SVETLANA POLTAVETS
EUGENE POLTAVETS

Guide to
Medicinal Mushrooms
of the Pacific Northwest

WARNING!

Consuming mushrooms is not recommended for people with increased sensitivity to mushrooms or who are intolerant to dishes made with mushrooms. Mushrooms should also not be consumed during pregnancy or while breast feeding.

To consume mushrooms safely, one must be able to distinguish between edible and poisonous species. If there is any doubt about the type of mushroom, please do not consume them. To apply any kind of fungi for medicinal purposes, it is always advisable to consult first with experts in this field.

The health advice presented in this book is intended only as an informative resource guide to help you make informed decisions; it is not meant to replace the advice of a physician or to serve as a guide to self-treatment. Always seek competent medical help for any health conditions or if there is any question about the appropriateness of a procedure or health recommendation. The publisher, employees and authors are not liable for the consequences of consuming mushrooms for medicinal purposes as presented in this book.

ISBN-13: 978-0-88839-351-7 [trade paperback]
ISBN-13: 978-0-88839-354-8 [epub]
Copyright © 2020 Svetlana & Eugene Poltavets

Library and Archives Canada Cataloguing in Publication

Title: Guide to medicinal mushrooms of the Pacific Northwest / Svetlana Poltavets,
Eugene Poltavets.
Other titles: Medicinal mushrooms of the Pacific Northwest
Names: Poltavets, Svetlana, author. | Poltavets, Eugene, author.
Description: Includes index.
Identifiers: Canadiana (print) 20190132906 | Canadiana (ebook) 20190132914 | ISBN
9780888393517
(softcover) | ISBN 9780888393548 (EPUB)
Subjects: LCSH: Edible mushrooms—Northwest, Pacific—Identification. | LCSH:
Fungi—Northwest,
Pacific—Identification. | LCSH: Medicinal plants—Northwest, Pacific—Identifica-
tion. | LCSH:
Mushrooms—Therapeutic use—Northwest, Pacific. | LCSH: Fungi—Therapeutic
use—Northwest, Pacific.
| LCGFT: Field guides.
Classification: LCC QK604.5 .P65 2019 | DDC 579.6/163209795—dc23

Illustrations and photographs are copyrighted by the artist or the Publisher.

Cover image: *Meripilus giganteus* by Michael Gäbler

Printed in the USA

PRODUCTION & DESIGN: E. Poltavets, M. Lamont, L. Raingam
EDITOR: M. MARTENS

We acknowledge the financial support of the Government of Canada through the Canada Book
Fund and the Canada Council for the Arts, and of the Province of British Columbia through the
British Columbia Arts Council and the Book Publishing Tax Credit.

Hancock House gratefully acknowledges the Semiahmoo, Kwantlen, Katzie &
Lummi First Nations, whose unceded traditional territories our offices reside upon.

Published simultaneously in Canada and the United States by

hancock

house

HANCOCK HOUSE PUBLISHERS LTD.
19313 Zero Avenue, Surrey, B.C. Canada V3Z 9R9
(604) 538-1114   Fax (604) 538-2262
HANCOCK HOUSE PUBLISHERS
#104-4550 Birch Bay-Lynden Rd, Blaine, WA, U.S.A. 98230-9436
(800) 938-1114   Fax (800) 983-2262
www.hancockhouse.com   sales@hancockhouse.com

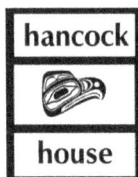

An enormous number of mushrooms types appear in the wild on the Pacific Coast. That variety exists due to the mild maritime climate. Scientists have long allocated fungi to a separate kingdom of living organisms. They appeared on Earth long before human beings and have played a huge role in human life. In addition to serving as food for humans and for many animals, birds and insects, they play an important role in nature and are actively involved in soil formation. They are employed in agriculture to assist in pest control. They have been used since ancient times as medicines and play an important part in many human industries: dairy, bakery, brewing, and winemaking, among others. They are an inexhaustible source of vitamins, trace elements, antibiotics and other medicines.

The role of fungi in human life systems is not fully understood, and scientists may yet discover many useful properties that can be utilized by humanity.

Since ancient times, mushrooms have been widely used in folk medicine. The treatment of diseases based on the use of medicinal mushrooms and drugs obtained from them is reffered to as fungotherapy. This method involves making decoctions, tinctures and various extracts that preserve the useful properties of the original organism. Fungi contain a large number of immuno-modulating substances that promote a speedy recovery. Mushrooms are rich in amino acids, minerals, plenty of vitamins, protein, fiber, lecithin, and other beneficial ingredients.

Of the nearly two hundred mushrooms included in this book, many, according to folk medicine and scientific research, can be used to enhance immunity, activate the body's defence systems and help prevent and treat malignant and benign tumours, or assist in the treatment of other diseases. Among this mushroom-rich part of the Earth are edible, conditionally edible, inedible, and poisonous mushrooms.

This manual does not provide a botanical description of fungi, only their distribution and fruiting time is indicated. More information to determine the type of fungus you have gathered can be found in the list of books to read. Also, this book doesn't provide recipes for using mushrooms for culinary purposes. It lists only the medicinal properties of mushrooms, used in traditional medicine and/or confirmed by scientific research. This information is not necessarily complete, as new research continues to update our knowledge. The purpose of this book is to draw the reader's attention to mushrooms not only as a healthy food but also as a source of natural medicinal substances that can assist in maintaining good health.

It's best never to touch mushrooms you do not know, because among them some may be deadly poisonous. For medicinal purposes, apply only those mushrooms that are recommended to you by specialists in this field: fungal therapists or traditional healers, who know the properties of mushrooms well.

While in the forest, enjoy the beauty, the fresh air and its gifts, treat it with respect and care. A frequent presence in nature has a beneficial effect on the nervous system and the human body as a whole.

Be healthy!

-- Svetlana & Eugene Poltavets

Additional Reading Material:
1. Mushrooms Demystified by David Arora, 1979
2. Growing Gourmet and Medicinal Mushrooms by Paul Stamets, 2000
3. Wild Edible Fungi: A Global Overview of Their Use and Importance to People by Eric Boa, 2005
4. The Fungal Pharmacy by Robert Rogers, 2011
5. Macromycetes: medicinal properties and biological characteristics by Solomon Vasser, 2012
6. Medicinal Mushrooms. Great Encyclopedia by Mikhail Vishnevsky, 2014
7. Compendium of Mycotherapy by Jan I. Lelley, Beate Berg, 2016
8. Healing Mushrooms: A Practical and Culinary Guide to Using Mushrooms for Whole Body Health by Tero Isokauppila, 2017
9. Medicinal Mushroom. Recent Progress in Research and Development. Edited by Dinesh Chandra Agrawal, Muralikrishnan Dhanasekaran, 2019
10. Medicinal Mushrooms of the Holarctic: anti-cancer and other therapeutic uses by Svetlana Poltavets, Eugene Poltavets (in publication, Hancock House)

ACKNOWLEDGEMENTS

We are grateful to everyone who helped us in finding and selecting the necessary information on medicinal mushrooms growing in the western part of Canada. Thanks to Hancock House for corrections and editorial guidance.

We also thank the specialists, pharmacologists, physicians and scientists who are currently working on creating medicines derived from fungi that may help cure cancer and other serious diseases.

We express our gratitude to the following professional and amateur photographers and web authors, the materials of which we used under the terms of their copyrights:

57 Andrews, Aarongunnar, A. Cortés-Pérez (Alonso), Adam Bryant (Ayedee), Agronomu.com, Ak ccm (Talk), Alan Rockefeller, Alden Dirks, Alexey Sergeev (Asergeev), AllanRz, Alok Mahendroo (Alok), Amatoxin Apocalypse, Andreas Eichler, Andreas Kunze, Andrei Yakimenko, Andrew C., Angelos Papadimitriou (Aggelos Xanthi), Ann B. (Ann F. Berger), Anna Baykalova (Anna_ru), Anneli Salo, Astro_al, Balkrishna, Becky (Beeker67), Björn S., BlueCanoe, Brian Adamo (Adamo588), Candicebshd.wordpress.com, Charles Sommer, Chmee2, Chris Cassidy (Cmcassidy), Chris Foss (The Vault Dweller), Christin (Ceanderz), Cindy Trubovitz (Trubo), Connor Adams (CLAdams), Dan Molter (Shroomydan), Dario Z. (Dario13), Dave W., David Tate, Davide Puddu, Doc850, Dperlstein, Eric Steinert, Erlon (Herbert Baker), Eva Skific (Evica), Eva Zupan, Evan Casey, Geoff Balme, George Chernilevsky, Gerhard Koller (Gerhard), Gillow2e, Glen van Niekerk (Primordius), Graco (Graceym99), Grzegorz "Spike" Rendchen, H. Krisp, Heather Waterman (Ripkord), Henk Monster, Herb (HerbM), Huafang, Ian Blaylock (Catfish Deity), Ian Dodd, Igor Yevdokimov, Igor Lebedinsky, I. G. Safonov (IGSafonov), Irene Andersson (Irenea), Jacob Kalichman (Pulk), Jay Pitts, Jason Alexander (J.A.), Jason Hollinger (Jason), JC (Dameeyola), JD (JD2), J-Dar, Jdx, Jean-Pol Grandmont, Jean Claude, Jensbn-commonswiki, Jerzy Opioła, Joe Mat, Jon Shaffer (Watchcat), Jörg Hempel, Josh Grefe (Mushme), Jsun Lau, Jymm, Kate Turner (Kathawk), Kruczy89, Len (Placeport), Len Worthington, Lucio Zibarova, Luke Smithson (Mycofreak), Mars 2002, Matt Welter (Mattfungus), Maynardjameskeenan, Meky, Michael Gäbler, Narodnymi.com, Norbert Nagel, Olga Kuznetsova, Patrick Harvey (Pg_harvey), Raphaël Blo, Rand Workman (Ranmofod), Rich Clark, Richard Bishop (Leciman), Ricky90501, Ringless Eschampignons, Ringless, Rob (Gourmand), Ron Pastorino (Ronpast), Ryane Snow (Snowman), Sasata, Sava Krstic (Sava), Schafhuber/pixelio.de, Sławomir Duda-Klimaszewski, SMoubray, Snow Morel, Speifensender, Sporulator, S. Rae, Stem2, Stro-bilomyces, Susanne Sourell (Suse), Szabi237, Tatiana Bulyonkova (Re-ssaure), Tatiana Svetlova, Terri Clements/Donna Fulton (Pinonbistro), Tim Sage (T. Sage), TNred, Tomaso Lezzi, Vesna Maric (Kalipso), Vlad Rotaru, Vladimir Briukhov, VMalikova, Walt Sturgeon (Mycowalt), Weed Lady (Sylvia), Wen Hsu (Qin2tang2), Włodzimierz Wysocki, Zaca, Zonda Grattus (Luridiformis), Σ64.

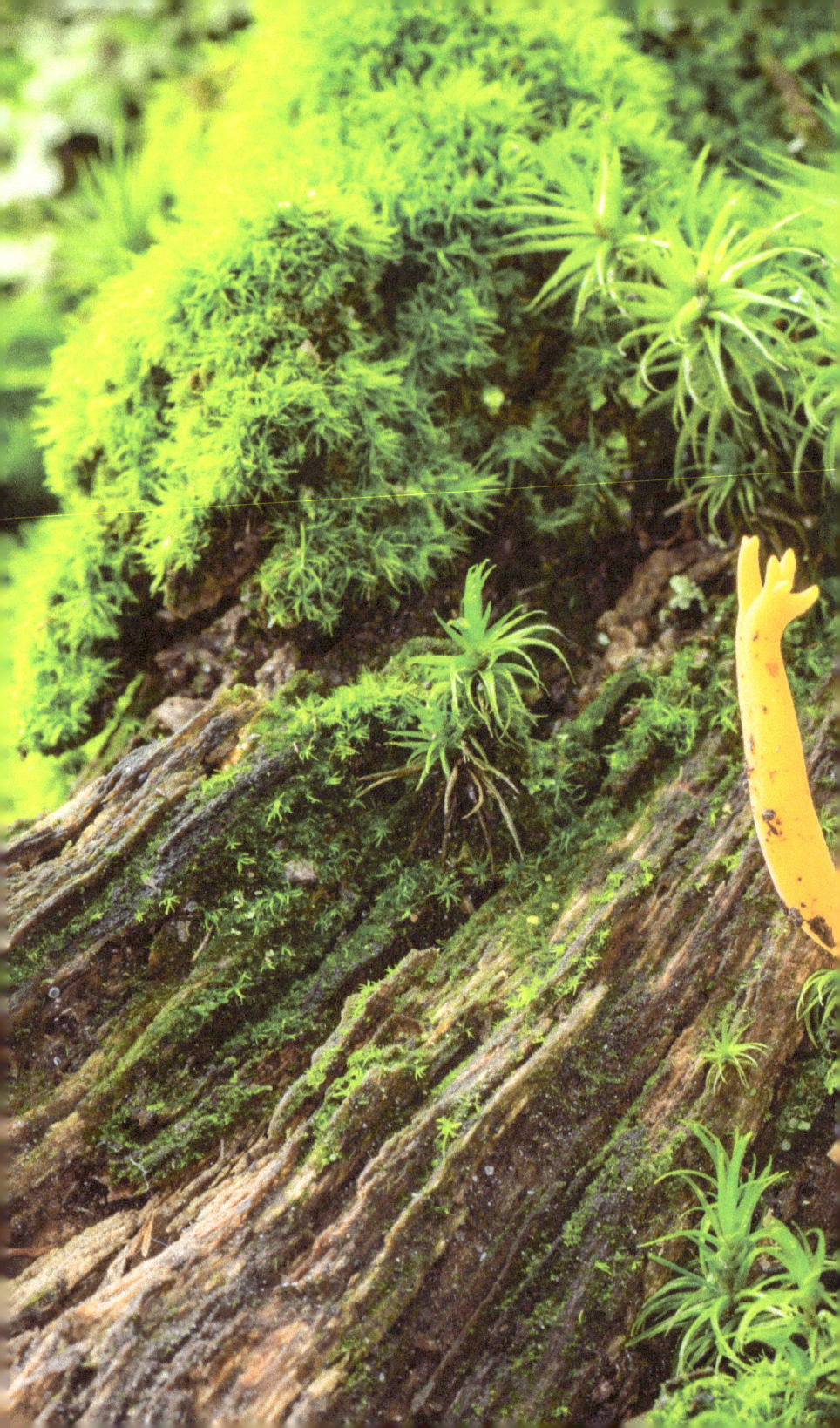

DEDICATIONS

This book is dedicated to our grandmother Ulyana Paramonov, a gifted and kind person who has always used natural means in her life and in housekeeping. Her knowledge and skills saved her life when she fell ill with breast cancer that developed after an accidental injury to her chest. She was strong in spirit, did not give up, independently cured herself with the folk remedies and lived a long, hardy and active life thereafter.

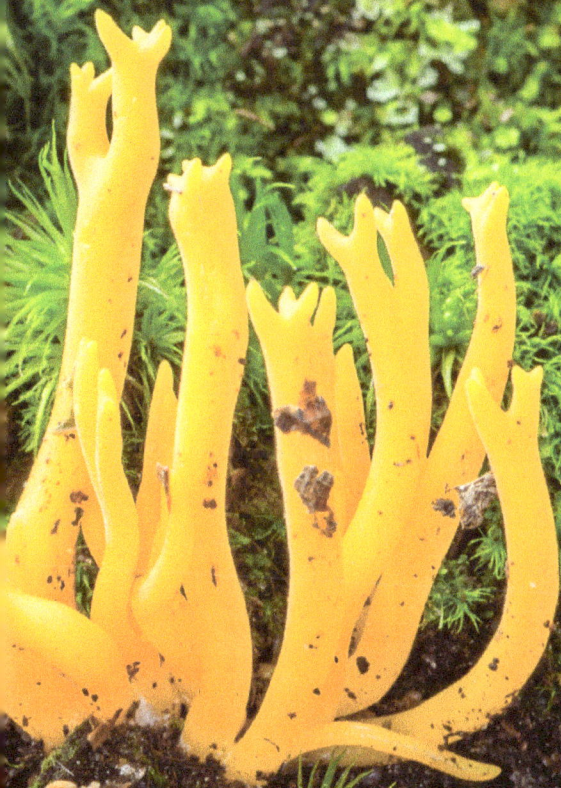

Agaricus albolutescens - Amber-Staining Agaricus

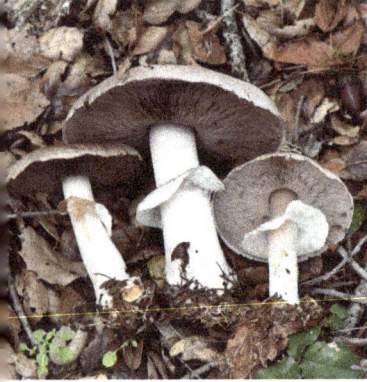

Edible. Grows in large numbers, either solitary or in groups, mostly under conifers in mountain areas or under oaks in mixed-forest mountainous areas. Season: August to September, in a warm climate from late autumn to early spring.

Medicinal uses: Strengthens and enhances the immune system, used to activate anti-tumor protective systems of the body and for the prevention and treatment of malignant tumors and benign formations.

Agaricus bisporus - Common Mushroom

Edible. Grows in large groups on manured areas, gardens, pastures, landfills, roadside ditches, on compost heaps. It is common under cypress but very rarely can be found in woods or on lawns. Season: May to late September, in a warm climate, year around.

Medicinal uses: Antibacterial and antiviral agent, used to treat diseases caused by Staphylococcus aureus (acne, impetigo, furunculus, phlegmon, carbuncles, staphylococcal burn-like skin syndrome, abscess, pneumonia, meningitis, osteomyelitis, endocarditis, infectious-toxic shock, sepsis), respiratory diseases, pulmonary tuberculosis, gastrointestinal and cardiovascular diseases, diabetes mellitus, colds and inflammatory diseases, provides an immuno-stimulating and immuno-modulating

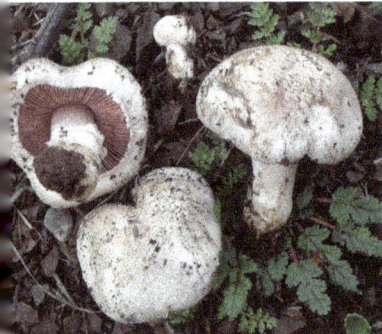

action, used to cleanse the body of toxins and remove heavy metals, improves brain functioning and enhances memory, treats allergy and asthma, typhus and paratyphoid, improves vision and strengthens the connective tissue in the body, used in gerontology, as it slows down the aging process, treats atherosclerosis, lowers cholesterol, improves the skin and mucous membranes, treats muscle pain, cramps, pain in the tendons, numbness of the limbs, lumbago, strengthens the nervous system.

Agaricus augustus - Prince of Mushrooms

Edible. It grows in deciduous, mixed and coniferous forests, in open woodland, and often occurs in groups or solitary near and on anthills. It appears in many places on rich organic soils, in disturbed places, along roads and streets, on flower beds, beneath trees in parks and gardens. Season: August to late October, in warm areas, year around.

Medicinal uses: Antibacterial agent, used for the treatment of diseases caused by Staphylococcus aureus (acne, impetigo, furunculus, phlegmon, carbuncles, staphylococcal burn-like skin syndrome, abscess, pneumonia, meningitis, osteomyelitis, endocarditis, infectious-toxic shock, sepsis), provides an immuno-stimulating and immuno-modulating action, treats typhus and paratyphoid, used in gerontology, as it reputedly slows down the aging process.

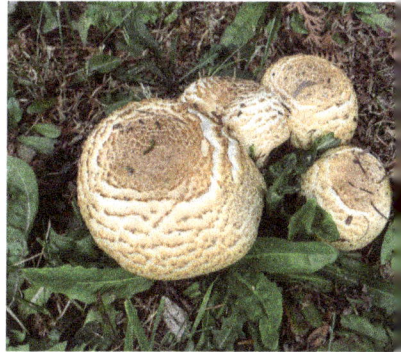

Agaricus bitorquis - Pavement Mushroom

Edible. It grows in many disturbed places in groups or rows on road shoulders, along streets, sidewalks, playgrounds, in parks. It can raise asphalt and even stones on the roadways. Season: May to October, in warm climate, year round.

Medicinal uses: Has antibacterial and antiviral effects, treats respiratory diseases. It is used for the treatment of diseases caused by Staphylococcus aureus. It protects the body against infections and inflammations, treats autoimmune diseases, allergies, bronchial asthma, diabetes mellitus, measles, arachnoiditis, convulsive syndrome, typhus and paratyphoid, obesity and cellulite. It provides an immuno-stimulating and immuno-modulating action, used to cleanse the body and for removal of heavy metals. It treats muscle pain, cramps, pain in the tendons, numbness of the limbs, lumbago. Used to strengthen the nervous system. It enhances hematopoiesis and treats diseases of the blood-vascular system. It normalizes the digestive system and lowers cholesterol. Can be used to improve skin condition and mucous membranes and in gerontology, as it slows down the aging process.

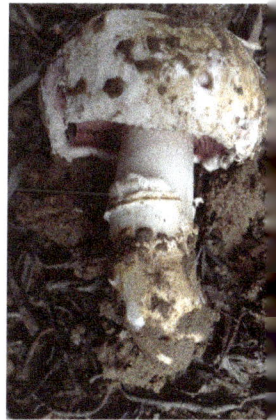

Agaricus campestris - Field Mushroom

Edible. Grows in humus-rich soil, in lawns, gardens, parks, cemeteries, vegetable gardens, in greenhouses, near housing and livestock farms, on pastures, fields, meadows, golf courses and on roadsides. Season: May to October, in warm climates, year round.

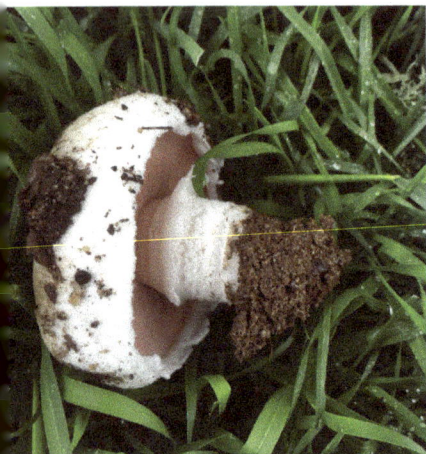

Medicinal uses: Has antibacterial effects, treats respiratory diseases, typhus and paratyphoid, pulmonary tuberculosis, diabetes 1 and 2, atherosclerosis, lowers cholesterol. It can be used to treat hypertension, heart pain, allergies, headaches, migraines, muscle pains, cramps, pain in the tendons, numbness of the limbs, lumbago. Treats wounds, burns. Used in gerontology, as it reputedly slows the aging process. It normalizes the digestive system, treats snake bites, and is effective in the last stages of oncology, helping patients cope with the disease.

Agaricus osecanus - Giant Horse Mushroom

Edible. Grows in large groups or rings in open woodland, in pastures, on lawns, in the shade of trees or shrubs where it won't be damaged by direct sunlight. It appears in many places on rich organic soils, along roads and streets, beneath trees in parks and gardens. Season: April to late October, in warm climates, year round.

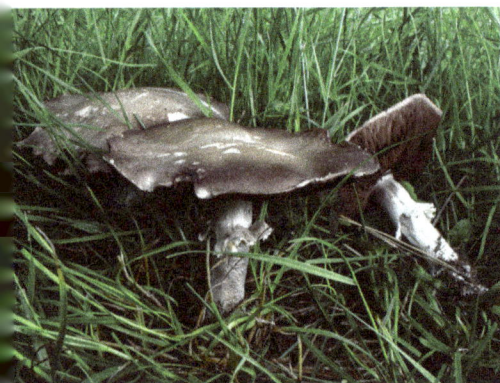

Medicinal uses: Provides an immuno-stimulating and immuno-modulating action. Used to lower cholesterol and to treat atherosclerosis and destroy cholesterol plaques. Strengthens and enhances the immune system, and is thought to activate anti-tumor protective systems of the body. Used for the prevention and treatment of benign formations and malignant tumors.

Agaricus semotus - Rosy Wood Mushroom

Edible. Grows in deciduous, coniferous and mixed forests, mainly with pines, spruce, larch, in open woodland, meadows and pastures, in virgin prairie, often occurs in groups or solitary. It appears along roadsides, on the edges of a mixed forest. In the forest it grows on a thick layer of leaf litter, on deadwood, on soil. Season: July to late November.

Medicinal uses: Strengthens and enhances the immune system, activates anti-tumor protective systems of the body, used for the prevention and treatment of malignant tumors, benign formations. It provides an immuno-stimulating and immuno-modulating action. Used to treat and prevent atherosclerosis, to lower cholesterol and destroy cholesterol plaques.

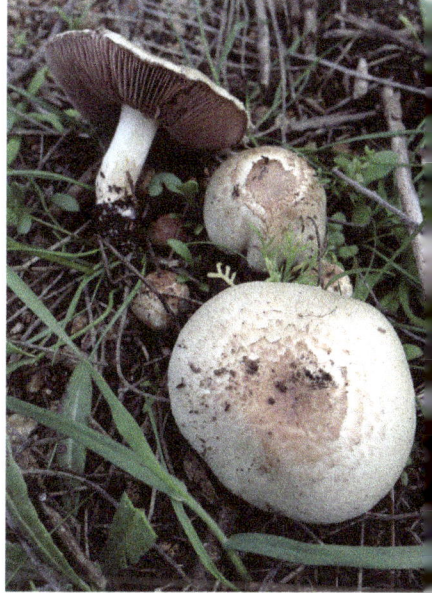

Agaricus silvaticus - Scaly Wood Mushroom

Edible. Grows in groups or solitary in mixed and coniferous forests, near and on anthills. Season: June to November.

Medicinal uses: Has antibacterial and antiviral effects, treats allergies, atherosclerosis, hypertension. Used to lower cholesterol, treat type 1 and 2 diabetes. Used to cleanse the body and remove heavy metals from it. The fungus treats measles, arachnoiditis and convulsive syndrome.
Srengthens the nervous system and slows down the aging process. It is used to improve the condition of the skin and mucous membranes, and to treat cellulite.

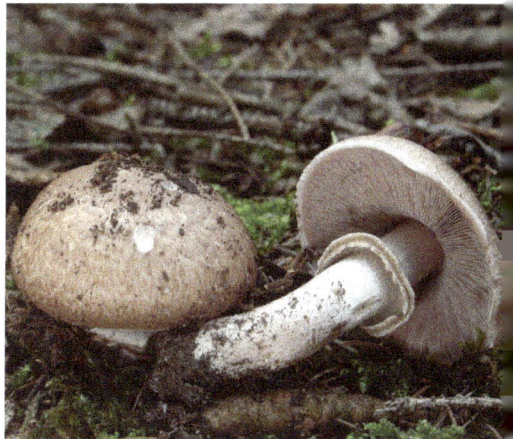

9

Agaricus subrufescens - Almond Mushroom

Edible. Grows in large groups or solitary in many places, on rich organic soils, along forest roads, on rotting leaves, at the borders between forest and field, in open woodland. Season: May to October.

Medicinal uses: Has antibacterial, antiviral and anti-fungal effects, treats type 1 and 2 diabetes, allergic reactions, bronchial asthma, atopic dermatitis, rhinitis, autoimmune diseases (polyarthritis, systemic lupus erythematosus, multiple sclerosis, scleroderma, etc.). It can be used to treat diseases of gastrointestinal tract, kidneys, liver, the urogenital system, blood and lymph, chronic hepatitis, cirrhosis. Reduces side effects of cancer surgery, radiation and chemotherapy. Helps regeneration of liver cells in cancer patients and removes poisons and toxins from the body. It strengthens the nervous system and treats nervous system exhaustion (depression, apathy, neuroses, fear, insomnia, etc.). It is used to treat chronic fatigue syndrome, and improves the condition and quality of life of critically ill patients. It treats encephalopathy and epilepsy, measles, arachnoiditis, convulsive syndrome. Contributes to the preservation of bone tissue, strengthens the body under severely stressful conditions. Slows down the aging process and improves condition of the skin and mucous membranes, treats cellulite. Can be used to treat impotency and restore male erection.

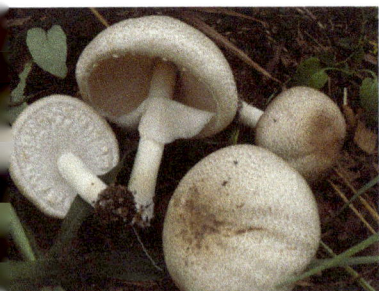

Agaricus subrutilenscens - Wine-colored Agaricus

Edible. Grows under trees in undisturbed deciduous, mixed and coniferous forests (alder, pine, redwood, Sitka spruce, oak), often occurs in small groups or solitary. Season: August to late October, in warm climates, year round.

Medicinal uses: Provides immuno-stimulating and immuno-modulating action, treats atherosclerosis, lowers cholesterol. Can be used for destruction of cholesterol plaques. Strengthens and enhances the immune system, activates anti-tumor protective systems of the body. Used for the prevention and treatment of malignant tumors and benign formations.

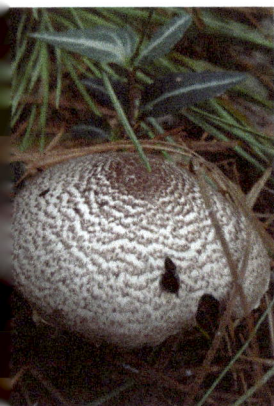

10

Agaricus xanthodermus - Yellow-Staining Mushroom

Poisonous. Grows in large groups or solitary, in mixed and deciduous forests (cypress, acacia, eucalyptus), in parks, meadows, pastures, on lawns, along roads and forest paths, orchards (olive) under trees. It differs from other Agaricus mushrooms as it has an unpleasant smell of carbolic acid, or iodine, or phenolic (unpleasant) odor, which causes a significant yellowing of the pulp at the base and where cut. Often it sits side-by-side with other edible species of mushrooms. Season: July to November, in warm climates, year round.

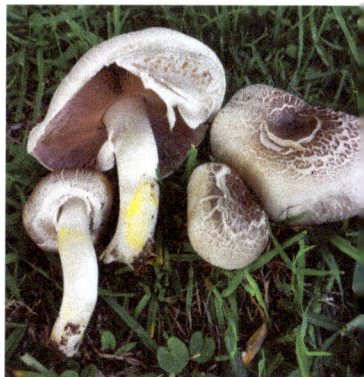

Medicinal uses: Has a strong antibacterial effect, treats diseases caused by gram-positive organisms and Salmonella spp. Can be used to treat food poisoning (including symptoms of vomiting and diarrhea), typhus and paratyphoid. It has a suppressing effect on hay bacillus, treats salmonellosis. It strengthens and enhances the immune system, activates anti-tumor protective systems of the body, and is used for prevention and treatment of benign formations and malignant tumors.

Albatrellus confluens - Polyporus Confluens

Edible. Grows in large groups on the ground among moss in mixed and coniferous forests of various types. It occurs mainly in mountain forests, rarely forms mycorrhiza with softwood trees. Season: July to October.

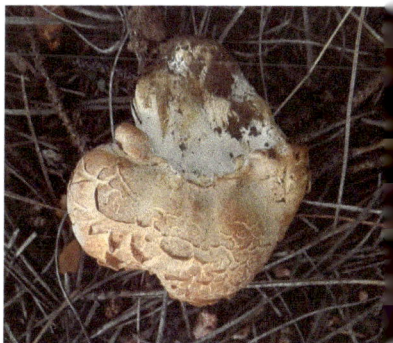

Medicinal uses: Has strong antibacterial effects, treats diseases caused by Staphylococcus aureus (acne, impetigo, boils, cellulitis, carbuncles, staphylococcal scalded skin syndrome, abcess, pneumonia, meningitis, osteomyelitis, endocarditis, toxic shock, sepsis), treats pulmonary tuberculosis. Has antioxidant and anti-inflammatory effects. Inhibits growth of gram-positive bacteria and hay bacillus. It reduces cholesterol in the blood and treats atherosclerosis. Has an analgesic effect.

Edible. Grows in deciduous and mixed forests, but prefer coniferous mountains of west coast of North America. Season: August to November.

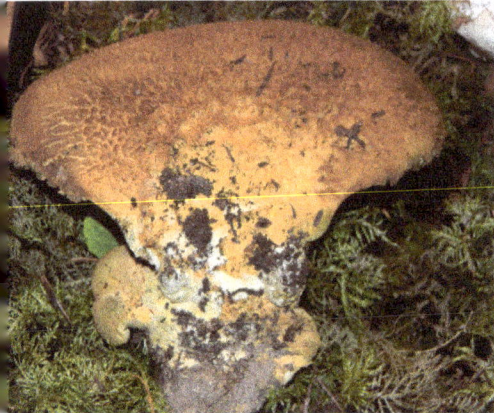

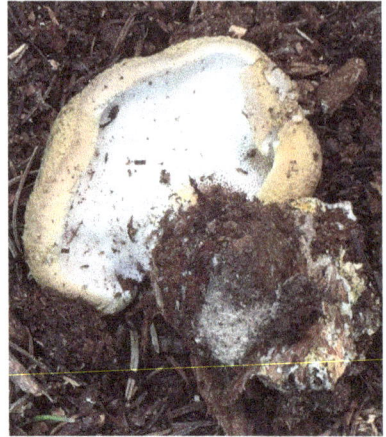

Medicinal uses: Has a strong antibacterial effect, treats pulmonary tuberculosis and diseases caused by Staphylococcus aureus. It can be used as a pain killer.

Edible. Grows in large inter-grown groups or solitary, in coniferous and mixed forests dominated by spruce, on glades, fringes, near roads, and also in mountains. It prefers neutral and alkaline soils, often grows in moss. Season: July to October.

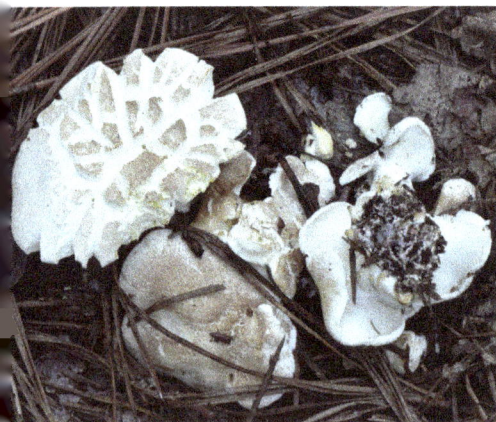

Medicinal uses: Has strong antibacterial and analgesic effects, treats pulmonary tuberculosis and diseases caused by Staphylococus aureus (acne, impetigo, furunculus, phlegmon, carbuncles, staphylococcal burn-like skin syndrome, abscess, pneumonia, meningitis, osteomyelitis, endocarditis, sepsis, infectious-toxic shock). It has antioxidant, anti-inflammatory and anti-fungal effects.

Edible. Grows on ground in deciduous and mixed forests, in parks, in gardens near trunks or stumps of lilac, willow, linden, alder. Often occurs alone or in small groups. It has a pleasant nutty taste and fleshy fruit body. Season: August to November.

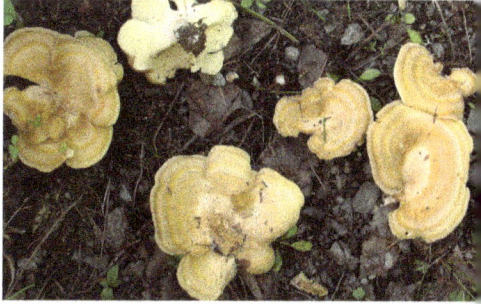

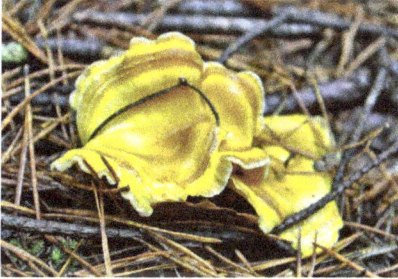

Medicinal use: Has an antibacterial effect. Strengthens and enhances the immune system, used to activate anti-tumor protective systems of the body. It can be used for the prevention and treatment of malignant tumors and benign formations.

Amanita caesarea - Caesar's Mushroom

Edible. A delicacy species. It grows in deciduous (oak, beech) and occasionally in coniferous forests, forming mycorrhiza with oak, beech, chestnut, less often with birch, hazel and other tree species. It prefers sandy soils, dry places. It fruits only on the southern slopes of the mountains on the fringes, glades, loves warm places. Season: July to October.

Medicinal uses: Has a strong antibacterial effect, treats diseases caused by Staphylococcus aureus (acne, impetigo, boils, cellulitis, carbuncles, staphylococcal scalded skin syndrome, abscess, pneumonia, meningitis, osteomyelitis, endocarditis, toxic shock, sepsis). It inhibits growth of hay bacillus.

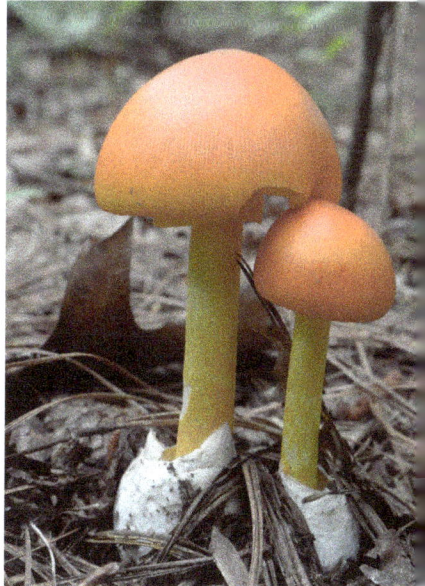

Inedible. It grows solitary or in large groups in coniferous, deciduous and mixed forests, in clearings and on open warm places with poor soils. The fungus prefers to grow near pines and oaks on sandy and slightly acidic soils. It forms mycorrhiza with birch, oak, pine and spruce. Occurs in the mountains to a height of 1400 metres. Season: July to November.

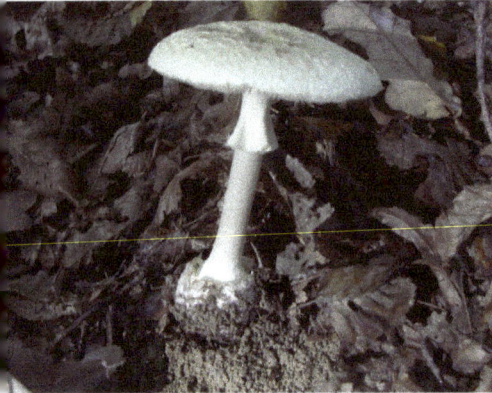

Medicinal uses: Has analgesic effects, treats non-healing wounds. Strengthens and enhances the immune system, activates anti-tumor protective systems of the body. Used for the prevention and treatment of malignant tumors and benign formations. Treats joint and skin diseases.

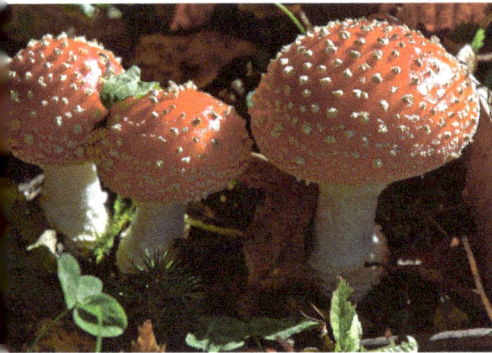

Conditionally edible. The fungus has long been classified as poisonous, but modern research shows that with proper preparation, it can be eaten. It needs to be boiled in water two to three times for 5 minutes, than drained. After that it can be cooked in dishes. Grows individually or in large groups throughout coniferous, deciduous and mixed forests, forming mycorrhiza with birch, spruce, pine and larch trees on all continents except Antarctica. It has a unique chemical composition and a range of positive effects on the human body. Season: August to October.

Medicinal uses: Has strong antibacterial, antiviral and anti-inflammatory effects, treats pulmonary and skin tuberculosis, treats diseases of the nervous system, neurological and psychiatric disorders (muscle cramps, "chorea," nervous excitement, intestinal and bladder

14

cramps, vascular spasms, congenital dementia, loss of coordination, solar pruritus, etc.) and restores lost memory. Helps with physical and mental fatigue and insomnia, treats diabetes mellitus and hypertension, enhances hematopoiesis. Has an analgesic effect (toothache, headache, heart pain) and is used for the treatment of muscle pain, seizures, pain in the tendons, numbness of the limbs, lumbago. It can be used to treat eye diseases: reduced vision, double vision, floaters, clouding of the lens and vitreous body, myopia, and inflammation of the eyelid edges. It treats benign prostatic hyperplasia and impotence, enhances libido both in men and women. Normalizes metabolism and can be used as a restorative agent. This is not yet a complete list of the medicinal properties of the fungus, which is being supplemented by ongoing research.

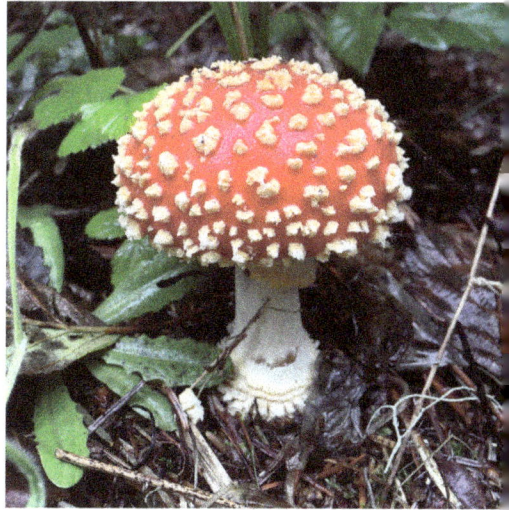

Amanita pantherina - Panther Cap

Inedible. Grows in deciduous (beech, oak), mixed and rarely in coniferous forests (pine), forming mycorrhiza with many trees. It can be found solitary or in large groups in meadows too. Season: July to October.

Medicinal uses: Has an antibacterial effect, treats non-healing wounds. Used to normalize and stimulate the body's metabolism. Used for the prevention and treatment of pain in the joints and bones. It strengthens and enhances the immune system, activates the anti-tumor protective systems of the body. Used for the prevention and treatment of benign formations and malignant tumors. The fungus is used to treat vascular diseases, atherosclerosis, and impotence.

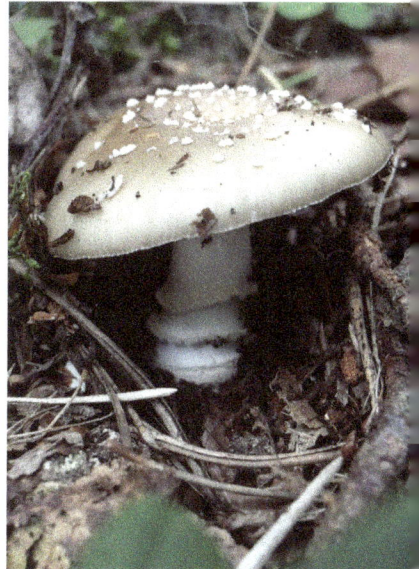

Amanita rubescens – Blusher

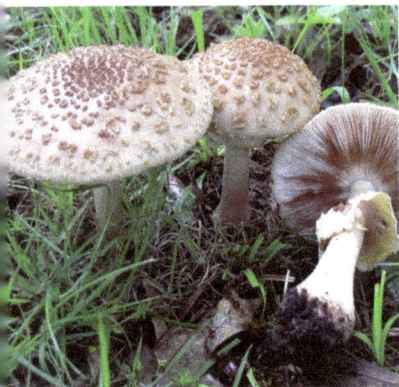

Edible. Grows solitary or in groups in deciduous and coniferous forests, forms mycorrhiza with birch and pine. Often this species is found along roads. Season: July to September.

Medicinal uses: Has strong antibacterial and antiviral effects, treats pulmonary tuberculosis and diabetes. It normalizes metabolism and treats obesity. It can be used to treat diseases of the nervous system and Alzheimer's disease.

Armillaria borealis - Northern Honey Fungus

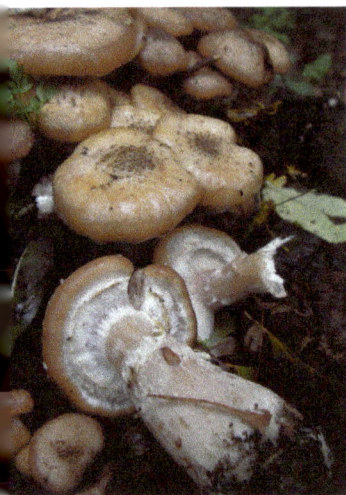

Edible. Fruiting bodies grow in bundles in deciduous and coniferous forests on living and dead trees. Cultivated on organic residues on an industrial scale in many countries. Season: late August to early winter, fructifies in large quantities in the first half of September.

Medicinal uses: Has strong antibacterial and anti-inflammatory effects, treats diabetes and diseases of the gastrointestinal tract. Strengthens lungs, heart, kidneys, stomach, liver. Has analgesic and sedative effects, treats joint diseases (arthrosis, arthritis, rheumatism, polyarthritis, osteochondrosis, psoriatic arthritis). It is used as an anesthetic for heart and headaches, treats muscle pain, cramps, pain in the tendons, numbness of the limbs, lumbago. It treats eye diseases (such as night blindness) and helps improve vision. It can be used to treat diseases of the nervous system (epilepsy, neurasthenia, dizziness, insomnia). It is used in gerontology, as it is said to slow down the aging process, and as a cosmetic agent: skin care, acne, wrinkles, rejuvenating facials, prevents dry skin. It has a tonic effect and stabilizes the overall state of the body, and helps with rehabilitation after a stroke. It has a protective effect against ionizing radiation. This is not yet a complete list of the medicinal properties of the fungus, which is being supplemented by scientific research.

Armillaria gallica - Bulbous Honey Fungus

Conditionally edible. These mushrooms need to be boiled once for 10 minutes in water, then drained, after which they can be used in various dishes. Grows in mixed forests, solitary or in small groups, on dead wood and roots, on rotting wood fragments (often preferring spruce and beech trees) and is more rarely found on ash, fir and other trees. It appears on rotting leaves or stumps, rarely occurs on dying trees. Season: end of August to beginning of winter.

Medicinal uses: Has strong antibacterial and anti-inflammatory effects, treats diseases caused by Staphylococcus aureus (acne, impetigo, boils, cellulitis, carbuncles, staphylococcal scalded skin syndrome, abscess, pneumonia, meningitis, osteomyelitis, endocarditis, toxic shock, sepsis). It has analgesic and sedative effects, helps to treat heartaches, headaches, muscle pain, cramps, pain in the tendons, numbness of the limbs, lumbago. It enhances hematopoiesis and treats cardiovascular diseases and hypertension, and lowers cholesterol. It can be used to treat diseases of the nervous system (epilepsy, neurasthenia, dizziness, insomnia) and joint diseases (arthrosis, arthritis, rheumatism, polyarthritis, osteochondrosis, psoriatic arthritis). It has a protective effect against ionizing radiation. It is used for the prevention and treatment of diabetes and for the production of protein bread made of the mycelial mass of Armillaria gallica for diabetics. It treats eye diseases (such as night blindness) and helps improve vision. Used in gerontology, as it is said to slow the aging process, and is used as a cosmetic agent (skin care, acne, wrinkles, rejuvenating facials), and to prevent dry skin. It helps with rehabilitation after a stroke. This is not yet a complete list of the medicinal properties of the fungus, which is being supplemented by the research of scientists.

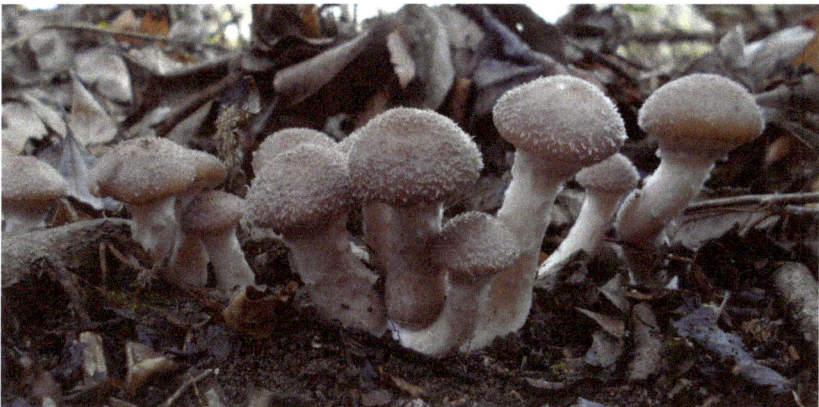

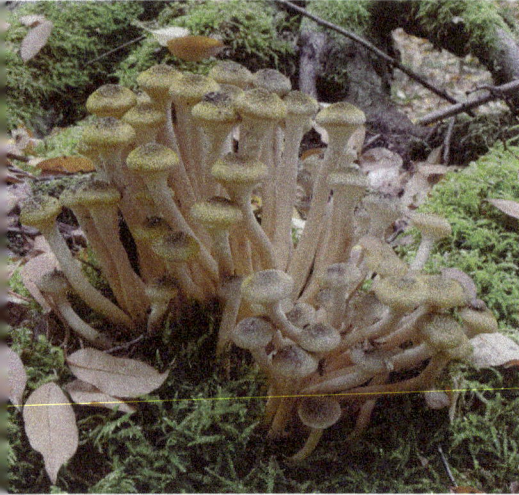

Edible. Grows in large groups in mixed forests on living and dead trees and on stumps, trunks, and roots. The fungus affects weakened trees of many species. Season: end of August to beginning of winter, it fruits a large amount in the first half of September.

Medicinal uses: Has strong antibacterial and anti-inflammatory effects, enhances hematopoiesis and is used for the treatment of cardiovascular diseases. It helps treat diseases of the nervous system (epilepsy, neurasthenia, dizziness, insomnia) and joint diseases (arthrosis, arthritis, rheumatism, polyarthritis, osteochondrosis, psoriatic arthritis). It has analgesic and sedative effects, helps to treat heartaches, headaches, muscle pain, cramps, pain in the tendons, numbness of the limbs, lumbago. Used for the prevention and treatment of diabetes and for the production of protein bread made of the mycelial mass of Armillaria mellea for diabetics. It treats eye diseases (such as night blindness) and helps improve vision. It is used for prevention and treatment of hypertension and to lower cholesterol. It has a tonic effect and stabilizes the overall state of the body. It is used in gerontology, as it is said to slow aging, and is used as a cosmetic agent (skin care, acne, wrinkles, rejuvenating facials) and to prevent dry skin. It has a protective effect against ionizing radiation and is used for rehabilitation after a stroke. Also treats rickets. This is not yet a complete list of the medicinal properties of the fungus, which is being supplemented by research.

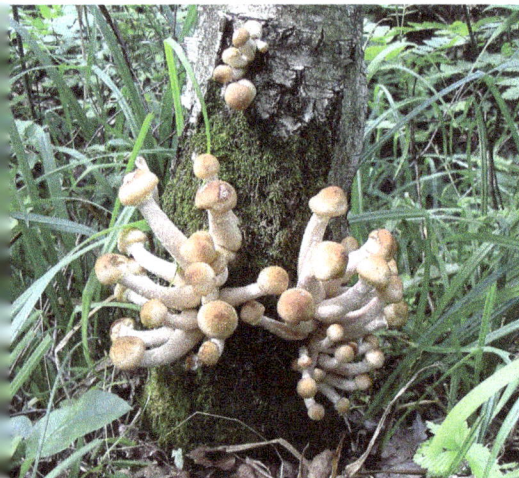

Edible. Grows in mixed and coniferous forests on the remains of rotting wood or at the base of the stumps and trunks of coniferous or hardwood trees. Season: end of summer until late autumn.

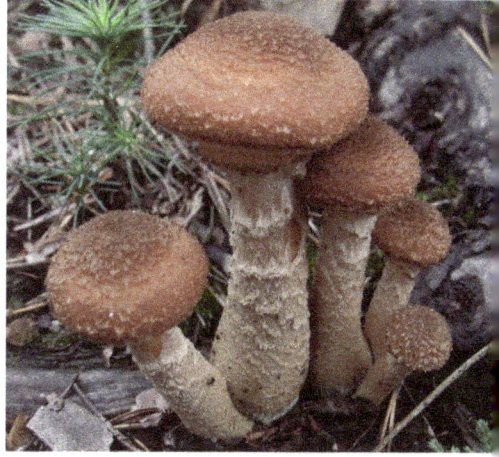

Medicinal uses: Has strong antibacterial and anti-inflammation effects, treats diseases caused by Staphylococcus aureus (acne, impetigo, boils, cellulitis, carbuncles, staphylococcal scalded skin syndrome, abscess, pneumonia, meningitis, osteomyelitis, endocarditis, toxic shock, sepsis). It has a protective effect against ionizing radiation and can be used for rehabilitation after a stroke. It treats diseases of the nervous system (epilepsy, neurasthenia, dizziness, insomnia) and joint diseases (arthrosis, arthritis, rheumatism, polyarthritis, osteochondrosis, psoriatic arthritis). Used for the prevention and treatment of diabetes and for the production of protein bread made of the mycelial mass of Armillaria ostoyae for diabetes patients. It enhances hematopoiesis and is used for the treatment of cardiovascular diseases, hypertension, and to lower cholesterol. It treats eye diseases (such as night blindness) and helps improve vision. It has a tonic effect and stabilizes the overall state of the body. It is used in gerontology, as it is said to slow down aging, and as a cosmetic agent (skin care, acne, wrinkles, rejuvenating facials). It helps prevent dry skin. It has analgesic and sedative effects, helps treat heartaches, headaches, muscle pain, cramps, pain in the tendons, numbness of the limbs, lumbago. It has a mild laxative effect. This is not yet a complete list of the medicinal properties of the fungus, which is being supplemented by scientific research.

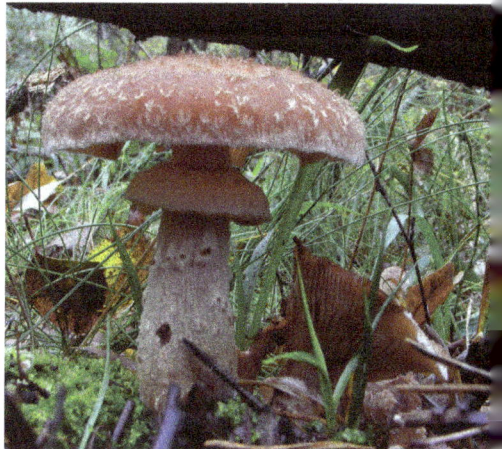

Edible. Grows in mixed and deciduous forests, in groups on trunks and stumps, on the plains, in mountainous regions, on the ground, sometimes as numerous colonies. Season: June to December.

Medicinal uses: Has strong antibacterial and anti-inflammatory effects, treats diseases caused by Staphylococcus aureus (acne, impetigo, boils, cellulitis, carbuncles, staphylococcal scalded skin syndrome, abscess, pneumonia, meningitis, osteomyelitis, endocarditis, toxic shock, sepsis), and has a suppressing effect on hay bacillus. Used for prevention and treatment of diabetes and for production of protein bread made of the mycelial mass of Armillaria tabescens for diabetes patients. It is used to treat diseases of the gastrointestinal tract and to strengthen lungs, kidneys, stomach, liver. It can be used to treat diseases of the nervous system (epilepsy, neurasthenia, dizziness, insomnia) and joint diseases (arthrosis, arthritis, rheumatism, polyarthritis, osteochondrosis, psoriatic arthritis). It has a protective effect against ionizing radiation and can used for rehabilitation after a stroke. It cures eye diseases (such as night blindness) and helps improve vision. It enhances hematopoiesis, used for the treatment of cardiovascular diseases, hypertension and to lower cholesterol. It used in gerontology, as it slows down the aging process and as a cosmetic agent (skin care, acne, wrinkles, rejuvenating facials), prevents dry skin. It has tonic effect and stabilizes the overall state of the body. It has an analgesic and sedative effects, helps treat heartaches, headaches, muscle pain, cramps, pain in the tendons, numbness of the limbs, lumbago. It has mild laxative effect. This is not yet a complete list of the medicinal properties of the fungus, which is supplemented by research of scientists.

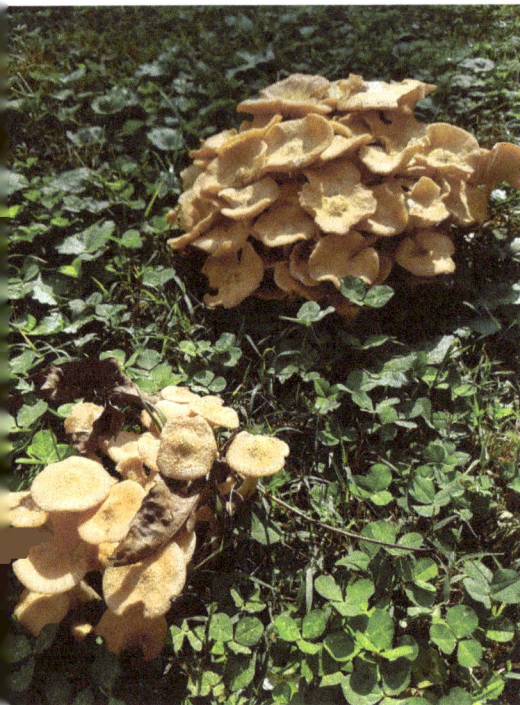

Auricularia auricula-judae - Wood Ear

Edible. It parasitizes on weakened or dead elderberry, alder and other deciduous trees. Usually it grows in small groups, but there are also single representatives. Season: all year round, but especially large harvest in autumn.

Medicinal uses: Has antibacterial and anti-inflammatory effects, treats respiratory system diseases. It removes toxins from the body and improves the composition of blood after chemotherapy. It enhances hematopoiesis and treats cardiovascular diseases (ischemic disease, hypertension), thrombosis, lowers cholesterol. It can be used to treat diabetes mellitus, obesity and cellulite. It has analgesic and hemostatic effects. Helps normalize the digestive system, removes and dissolves stones in the gallbladder and kidneys. It is used in gerontology, as it is said to slow down the aging process. It has anti-mutagenic and tonic effects and can be used to treat allergies.

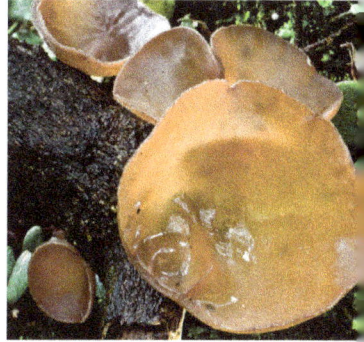

Auricularia mesenterica - Tripe Fungus

Edible. It grows in deciduous, mostly lowland forests on fallen tree trunks, on stumps of elm, poplar, ash and other species. The mushroom can be found sometimes on weakened fruit trees in gardens. Season: all year round, and in autumn it bears more fruit.

Medicinal uses: Has anti-inflammatory and antibacterial properties, and also has anti-ulcer effect. It provides an immuno-stimulating and immuno-modulating action. It activates anti-tumor protective systems of the body, strengthens and enhances the immune system. Used for prevention and treatment of malignant tumors and benign formations. It treats food poisoning. It contributes to the dissolution of stones in the gallbladder and kidneys. It can be used for to help normalize blood sugar and cholesterol. It has an anti-allergic effect, so it is used to treat allergies of various origin.

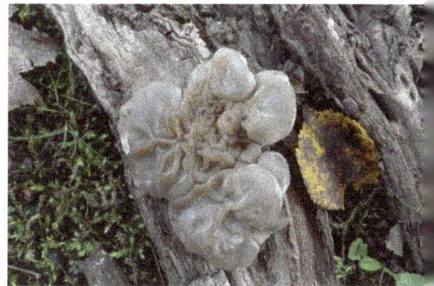

Boletus aereus - Dark Cep

Edible. Grows mostly in deciduous and mixed forests (beech, oak, hornbeam, pine), solitary or in groups. It prefers humus-rich soil. Season: May to October.

Medicinal uses: Has antibacterial, antiviral and anti-inflammatory effects, treats pulmonary tuberculosis, suppresses the activity of influenza and HIV viruses. It removes toxins from the body, inhibits the growth of cancer cells and the growth of metastases. It can be used to treat cardiovascular and lymphatic systems diseases, improves hematopoiesis. It has an analgesic effect and treats headaches, muscle pain, seizures, pain in the tendons, numbness of the limbs, lumbago. It normalizes the digestive system and treats gastrointestinal diseases. It treats burns, persistent ulcers, bruises, frostbite. Can be used to treat impotence and improve sexual desire. It increases vitality and speeds up metabolism.

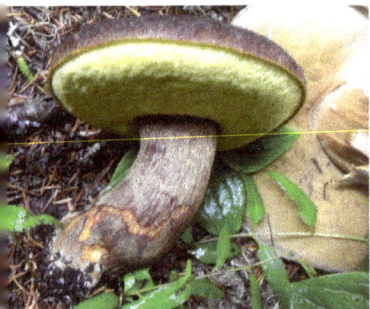

Boletus badius - Bay Bolete

Edible. Grows solitary or in groups, mainly in coniferous and mixed forests on glades and clearings, on litter, on sandy soils and in moss, at the base of trees, in lowlands and mountains. Can be found in small groups on stumps, under white pine, spruce, beech, birch, oak, chestnut and other trees. Season: June to November.

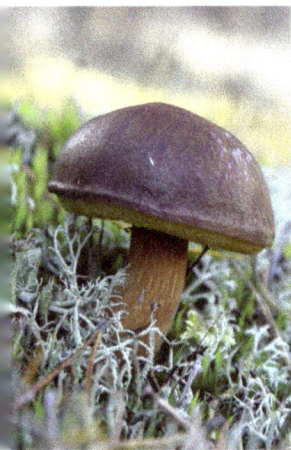

Medicinal uses: It inhibits the growth of cancer cells and the growth of metastases. It has a sedative effect and is used to treat headaches. It helps to remove toxic substances from the body. Used to treat cardiovascular diseases (angina pectoris), hypertension and gastrointestinal diseases. It suppresses the activity of influenza and HIV viruses. It has an antioxidant effect, improves vitality and speeds up metabolism. It treats burns, bruises, frostbite and persistent ulcers, obesity and cellulite. It strengthens and enhances the immune system, activates anti-tumor protective systems of the body. Used for the prevention and treatment of benign formations (cysts, broids) and malignant tumors.

22

Boletus edulis - Penny Bun

Edible. One of the best edible mushrooms, it grows solitary or in groups in coniferous and mixed forests, in meadows, glades, forest plantations, on stumps, forming mycorrhiza with various trees (pine, spruce, beech, birch, oak, etc.). Season: late May to October.

Medicinal uses: Has antibacterial, antiviral and anti-inflammatory effects, suppresses the activity of influenza and HIV viruses. Helps to remove toxic substances from the body, inhibits the growth of cancer cells and the growth of metastases. It has an analgesic effect and treats headaches, muscle pain, seizures, pain in the tendons, numbness of the limbs, lumbago. Used for prevention and treatment of cardiovascular (angina pectoris) and lymphatic system diseases, enhances hematopoiesis. It normalizes the digestive system and treats gastrointestinal diseases. It treats burns, bruises, frostbite, persistent ulcers and skin diseases (dermatitis). It improves vitality and speeds up metabolism, treats impotence and helps restore sexual desire. Used in gerontology, as it is said to slow down the aging process, used as a cosmetic agent (skin care, acne, wrinkles) and to improve the skin and mucous membranes.

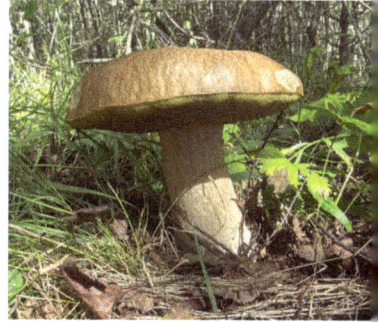

Boletus felleus (Tylopilus felleus) - Bitter Bolete

Conditionally edible. Grows in small groups or solitary in coniferous and mixed forests, often under birches and oaks, in the crevices of old trees, under fallen pine trunks, and on rotten stumps. The mushroom is very bitter, and this bitterness does not go away with soaking and boiling. The mushroom is suitable only for drying, in which case the bitterness completely disappears. It forms mycorrhiza with coniferous and deciduous trees. Season: June to October.

Medicinal uses: Has antibacterial effects and treats acne in adolescents. It restores liver cells after damage. It provides an immuno-stimulating and immuno-modulating action. Strengthens and enhances the immune system and activates the body's anti-tumor protective systems. Has a choleretic effect. Used to prevent and treat malignant tumors and benign formations.

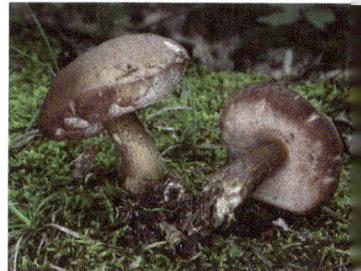

23

Boletus reticulatus - Summer Cep

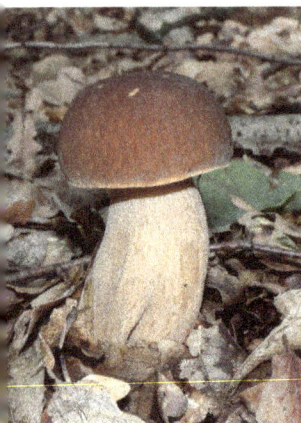

Edible. Grows solitary or in groups on edges and clearings in light deciduous forests. Prefers dry, alkaline soils. It forms mycorrhiza predominantly with trees of the Betulaceae family (beech, oak, chestnut) and hornbeam. Season: late May to October.

Medicinal uses: Has antibacterial and anti-inflammatory effects (abscesses, furunculosis), suppresses the activity of influenza and HIV viruses. It inhibits the growth of cancer cells and the growth of metastases, helps to remove toxic substances from the body, improves vitality and speeds up metabolism. It treats impotence and helps improve sexual desire. Used to treat cardiovascular (angina pectoris) and gastrointestinal diseases, and normalize the digestive system. It enhances hematopoiesis and is used to treat diseases of the lymphatic system. Used in gerontology, as it is said to slow down the aging process, and as a cosmetic agent (skin care, acne, wrinkles, anti-aging, etc.). Used to treat headaches, muscle pain, seizures, pain in the tendons, numbness of the limbs, lumbago, burns, bruises, frostbite and persistent ulcers, skin diseases (dermatitis).

Boletus rex-veris - Spring King Bolete

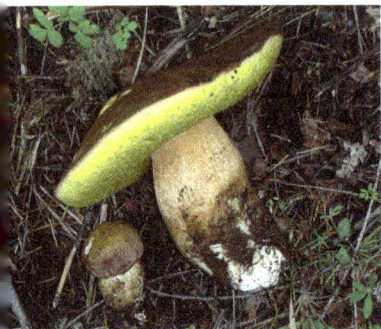

Edible. Grows solitary or in groups in coniferous and mixed mountain forests, forming mycorrhiza with pine (Pinus ponderosa, Pinus contorta subsp. murrayana), firs (Abies concolor and Abies species), and other evergreen trees. It is a common late-spring mountain bolete. Can be found in the mountains at an altitude of up to 2000m. Season: May to July.

Medicinal uses: Strengthens and enhances the immune system, activates anti-tumor protective systems of the body. Used for the prevention and treatment of malignant tumors and benign formations.

Calocera viscosa - Yellow Stagshorn

Edible. Grows solitary or in groups on the ground, on dying pine trunks, on roots, in moss, on the woody remains of coniferous trees, forest edges, and clearings. Season: July to October.

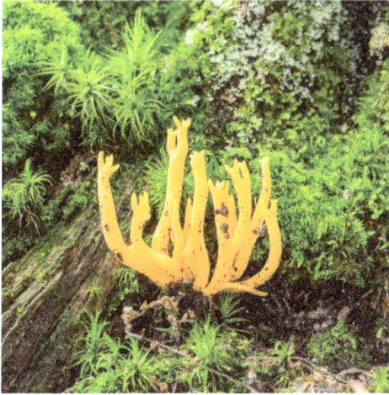

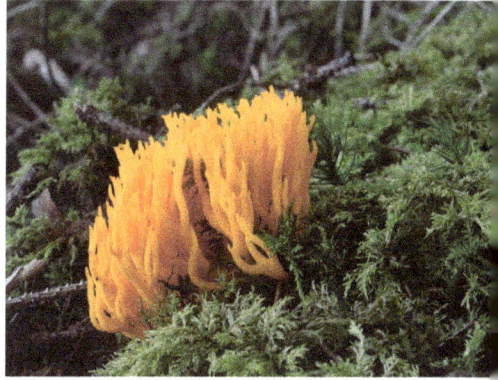

Medicinal uses: Strengthens the immune system, activates anti-tumor protective systems of the body. Used for the prevention and treatment of malignant tumors and benign formations.

Calocybe gambosa - St. George's Mushroom

Edible. It grows solitary or in groups, sometimes forming huge "fairy rings" in fields, meadows, forests, on roadsides, pastures, forest edges, and on open fertilized places. Season: March to July.

Medicinal uses: Has an antibacterial effect, suppresses hay bacillus, treats tuberculosis and diabetes mellitus. It has analgesic effects and treats migraines. It has a beneficial influence on the brain, used to stimulate the removal of heavy metals and toxins from the body. Strengthens the bones, normalizes body metabolism, treats chronic fatigue. Used as a restorative remedy.

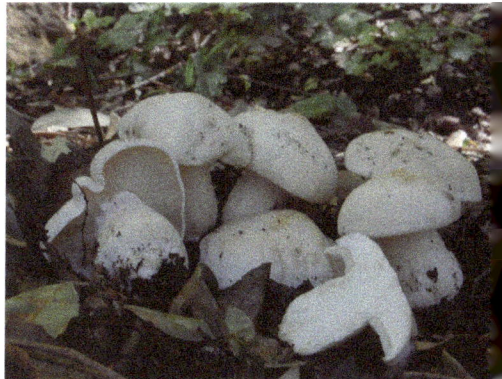

Calvatia gigantea - Giant Puffball

Edible when young. It grows in moist deciduous and mixed forests, solitary or in large groups in the grass, in the moss, on roadsides, along the edges of ditches, in gardens, parks, grasslands, prairies, in mountainous areas. Season: July to October.

Medicinal uses: Has antibacterial, anti-inflammatory and antimutagenic effects, treats pulmonary tuberculosis, bronchial asthma, respiratory diseases. It helps to remove and dissolve stones in the gallbladder and kidneys, and is used to treat of gastrointestinal and kidney

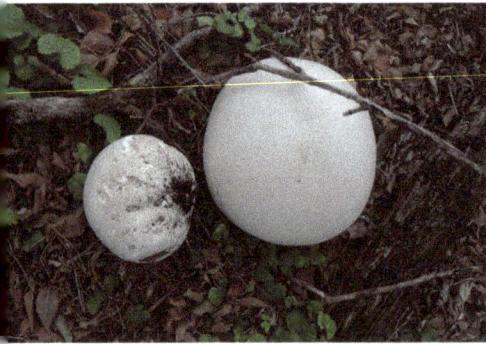

diseases. It has analgesic and anti-pyretic effects, treats diseases of the endocrine glands and lymphatic system (sarcoidosis). It has hemostatic and antitoxic effects. It can be used to treat cardiovascular diseases and hypertension. It has anti-fungal and wound-healing effects, used for the treatment of hives and smallpox. It strengthens the reproductive organs.

Calvatia utriformis - Mosaic Puffball

Edible when young. It grows solitary or in small groups on forest edges, glades and open areas on sandy soils that are in deciduous and mixed forests. Season: July to November.

Medicinal uses: Has strong antibacterial and antiviral effects, inhibits the activity of influenza and HIV viruses. It treats diseases caused by Staphylococcus aureus (acne, impetigo, boils, cellulitis, carbuncles, staphylococcal scalded skin syndrome, abscess, pneumonia, men-

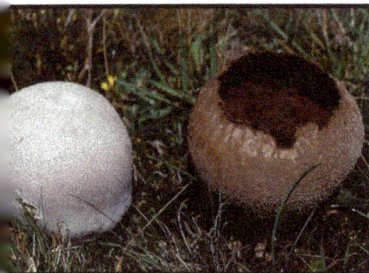

ingitis, osteomyelitis, endocarditis, toxic shock, sepsis), enteritis and cystitis, intestinal, paroxysmal and septic escherichiosis. It is used for the treatment of angina, acute glomerulonephritis and rheumatism. It treats kidneys, skin diseases and non-healing wounds, salmonellosis. It is used for strengthening the organs of the reproductive system.

Cantharellus cibarius - Golden Chanterelle

Edible. Grows in coniferous and mixed forests, forming mycorrhiza with various species of trees, often with oak, beech, birch, pine, and spruce trees. It can be found solitary or in large groups among the grass, wet moss, under fallen leaves. Golden Chanterelle differs from other similar fungi because it practically never contains worms and insect larvae in the pulp. Season: June to December.

Medicinal uses: Has antibacterial, antiviral, and anti-inflammatory effects, treats respiratory diseases. It has strong antihilmintic effect (enterobiosis, teniosis, trichocephalus, ascariasis, nematodes, giardiasis, schistosomiasis, opisthorchiasis, clonorchiasis, pinworms, cysticercosis). It treats intestinal lambliasis and skin diseases. Used to treat pulmonary tuberculosis and liver cirrhosis, fatty hepatosis, hemangiomas, and hepatitis C. It is used for the treatment of eye diseases, improves reduced vision, treats "night blindness". Treats circulatory system diseases and enhances hematopoiesis. It regulates fat metabolism, used for weight loss. It removes toxins from the body and improves general condition and tone.

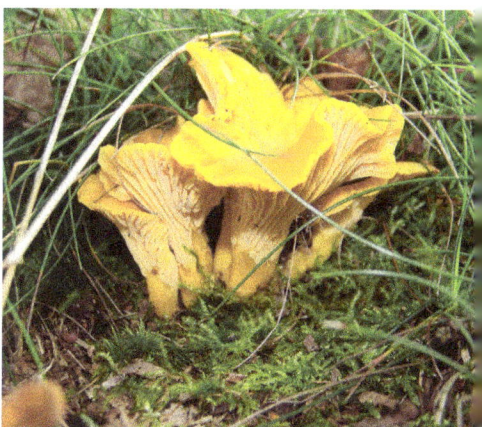

Catathelasma imperiale - King Mushroom

Edible. Can be found in mixed and coniferous (spruce) forests, in mountainous areas at high altitudes. It prefers to grow on calcareous soils. Season: July to October.

Medicinal uses: Enhances the immune system. Used to activate anti-tumor protective systems of the body. It can be used for the prevention and treatment of malignant tumors and benign formations.

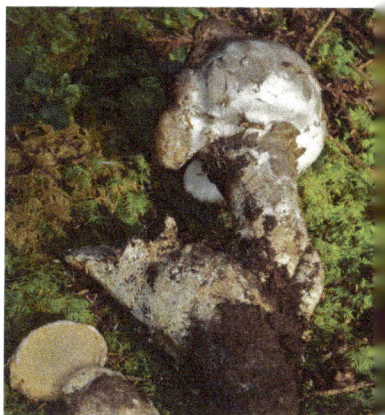

Cerrena unicolor - Mossy Maze Polypore

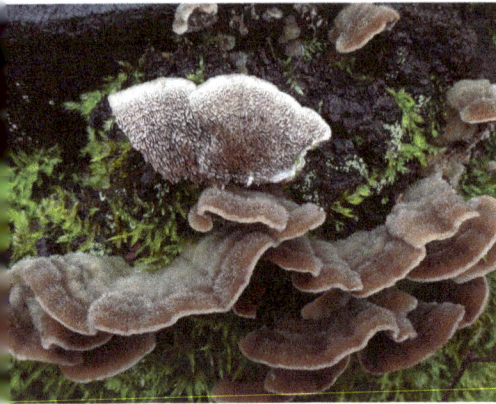

Inedible. Grows on dead stumps and thick branches of many deciduous species (birch, alder), near roads, on glades throughout the Northern Hemisphere. Dry last year's bodies are found in the spring. Season: from June to October.

Medicinal uses: Has an antiviral effect, strengthens and enhances

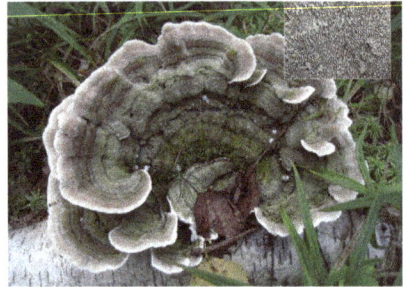

the immune system, activates anti-tumor protective systems of the body. Can be used for the prevention and treatment of malignant tumors and benign formations.

Clavaria purpurea - Purple Coral

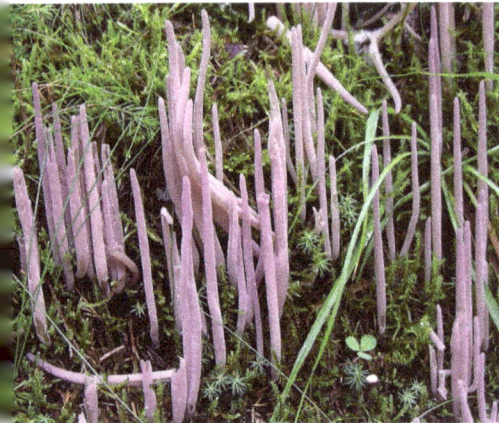

Edible. Grows in small or large groups on the remains of decaying wood, leaf litter, and among moss in mixed and coniferous forests of various types. Fruit bodies grow in the form of bushes, collected in small piles, the colour may be purple, grayish-purple, smoky brown with a purple hue, less often pale. Season: July to October.

Medicinal uses: Can be used to treat mental diseases and neuroses. It has an analgesic effect and treats headaches and migraines. Used for the stimulation of difficult births, incomplete abortion, atony of the uterus, and stimulation of uterine contractions. Treats hypertension.

Edible when fresh and young. Grows in small groups or solitary on wood waste, decaying wood, in moss and in grass in deciduous and coniferous forests. The fruiting body of the fungus is bushy, with long vertical branchlets, yellowish-ocher color with a pinkish tint, and crowned toothed tips. Season: April to September.

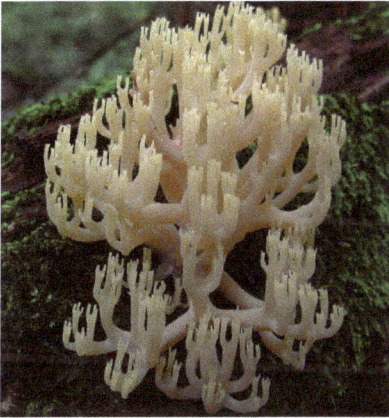

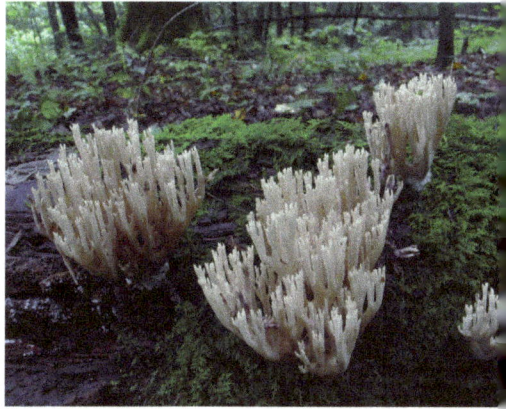

Medicinal uses: Strong antibacterial effect. It treats diseases caused by Staphylococcus aureus (acne, impetigo, boils, cellulitis, carbuncles, staphylococcal scalded skin syndrome, abscess, pneumonia, meningitis, osteomyelitis, endocarditis, toxic shock, sepsis) and is able to fight resistant forms of staphylococcus.

Conditionally edible. Grows solitary or in small groups in coniferous forests, often found on wood debris. Season: September to October.

Medicinal use: Strengthens and enhances the immune system, activates anti-tumor protective systems of the body. Used for the prevention and treatment of benign formations and malignant tumors.

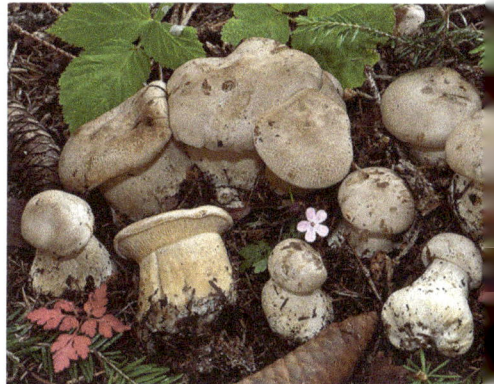

Clitocybe gibba - Common Funnel

Edible. Grows in small groups, rarely solitary, under deciduous trees in leaf litter. These mushrooms are common in forests of various types. They can be found along the roads, in rough grass or heaths. Season: July to September.

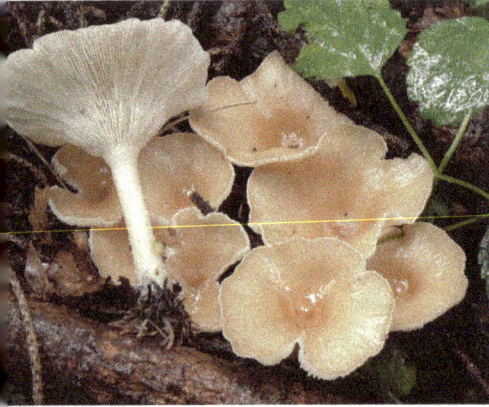

Medical uses: Strengthens and enhances the immune system, activates anti-tumor protective systems of the body. Can be used for the prevention and treatment of malignant tumors and benign formations. Removes accumulated slags, salts and heavy metals, toxins from the body. It lowers cholesterol, prevents blood clots, treats respiratory diseases. It can be used to prevent and treat urolithiasis.

Clitocybe clavipes - Club-footed Clitocybe

Conditionally edible. When combined with alcohol, it is poisonous. Usually grows solitary or in small groups in coniferous, mixed and deciduous forests. In the period of active fruiting, it appears very abundantly and in large groups. Out of the coniferous trees, this fungus prefers pine, and out of the deciduous types, it will mostly likely be found around birch trees. Season: mid-July to November.

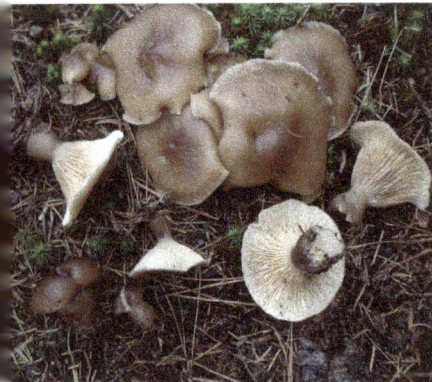

Medicinal uses: Has antibacterial and anti-fungal effects. It treats alcohol dependence. It has a suppressing effect on hay bacillus, treats food poisoning (including vomiting and diarrhea symptoms). Can be used for the treatment of tuberculosis. It treats epilepsy. Strengthens the immune system and activates anti-tumor protective systems of the body. Used to prevent and treat malignant tumors and benign formations.

Clitocybe fragrans - Fragrant Funnel

Edible. Grows in groups, rarely solitary, under deciduous and coniferous trees. The mushroom has a distinct anise smell. Season: May to September.

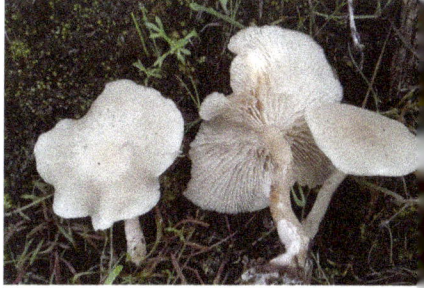

Medical uses: Has a strong antibacterial effect, treats diseases caused by Staphylococcus aureus (acne, impetigo, boils, cellulitis, carbuncles, staphylococcal scalded skin syndrome, abscess, pneumonia, meningitis, osteomyelitis, endocarditis, toxic shock, sepsis). Used to treat respiratory diseases and pulmonary tuberculosis. It lowers cholesterol and treats kidney stones. The mushroom can help in the treatment of epilepsy. It strengthens the immune system and activates anti-tumor protective systems of the body. Used for the prevention and treatment of malignant tumors and benign formations.

Clitocybe geotropa - Trooping Funnel

Edible. It grows in groups, in rows, or forming "fairy circles" in deciduous and mixed forests. Can be found by forest roadsides, grassy meadows, and in bushes. Season: July to end of October.

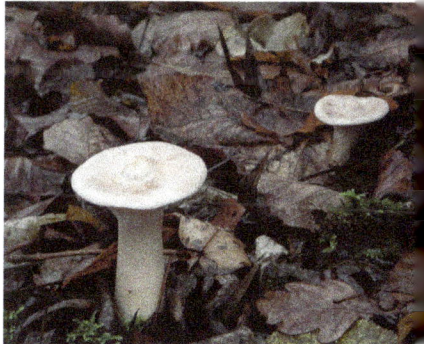

Medicinal uses: Has strong antibacterial effects, treats diseases caused by Staphylococcus aureus (acne, impetigo, boils, cellulitis, carbuncles, staphylococcal scalded skin syndrome, abscess, pneumonia, meningitis, osteomyelitis, endocarditis, toxic shock, sepsis). Can be used for the treatment of typhoid, paratyphoid, pulmonary tuberculosis, brucellosis, food poisoning (including vomiting and diarrhea symptoms). It has a suppressing effect on hay bacillus. Can be used for the treatment of epilepsy. It strengthens the immune system and activates anti-tumor protective systems of the body. Used for the prevention and treatment of malignant tumors and benign formations.

Clitocybe maxima - Large Funnel Cap

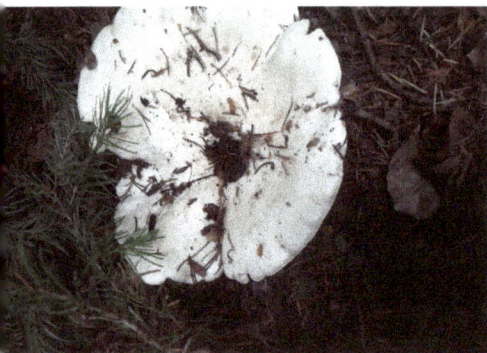

Conditionally edible. Grows in groups, in rows, or forming "fairy circles" in deciduous and mixed forests. It can be found by forest roadsides, grassy meadows. Season: July to late October.

Medicinal uses: Has strong antibacterial effects, treats diseases caused by Staphylococcus aureus (acne, impetigo, boils, cellulitis, carbuncles, staphylococcal scalded skin syndrome, abscess, pneumonia, meningitis, osteomyelitis, endocarditis, toxic shock, sepsis). Can be used for the treatment of pulmonary tuberculosis and epilepsy. It has antioxidant activities. The fungus reduces high levels of cholesterol. Strengthens the immune system, activates anti-tumor protective systems of the body. Used for the prevention and treatment of malignant tumors and benign formations.

Clitocybe nebularis - Clouded Agaric

Conditionally edible. Grows throughout the coniferous (spruce) and mixed (with birch, oak, fir) forests, often forming long lines and "fairy rings." Season: middle of August to end of November.

Medicinal uses: Has strong antibacterial and anti-fungal effects, treats diseases caused by Staphylococcus aureus (acne, impetigo, boils, cellulitis, carbuncles, staphylococcal scalded skin syndrome,

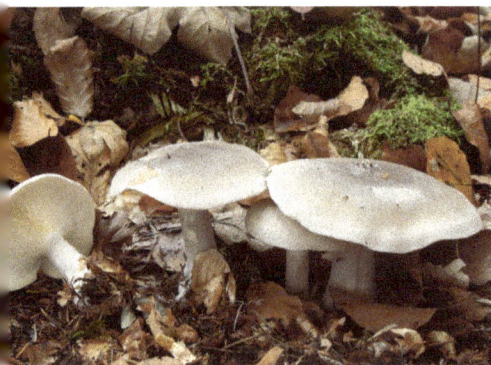

abscess, pneumonia, meningitis, osteomyelitis, endocarditis, toxic shock, sepsis). Can be used for the treatment of pulmonary tuberculosis and candidiasis (thrush). It can treat epilepsy. It strengthens the immune system, activates the anti-tumor protective systems of the body. Used for the prevention and treatment of malignant tumors and benign formations.

Clitocybe odora - Aniseed Toadstool

Edible. Can be found on wood debris in coniferous and deciduous forests. Season: July to September.

Medicinal uses: Has a strong antibacterial effect, treats diseases caused by Staphylococcus aureus (acne, impetigo, boils, cellulitis, carbuncles, staphylococcal scalded skin syndrome, abscess, pneumonia, meningitis, osteomyelitis, endocarditis, toxic shock, sepsis). Can be used for the treatment of pulmonary tuberculosis and epilepsy. It strengthens the immune system, activates anti-tumor protective systems of the body. Used for the prevention and treatment of malignant tumors and benign formations.

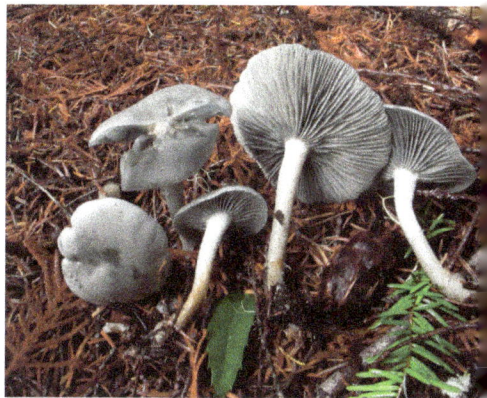

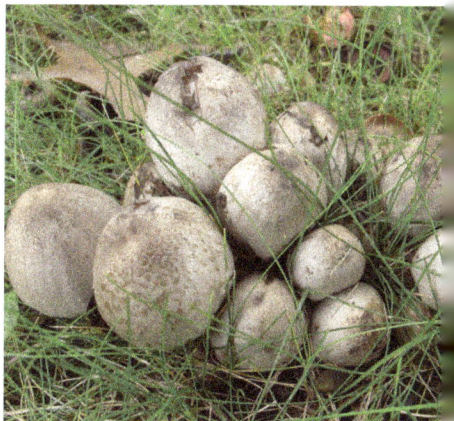

Coprinus atramentarius - Common Ink Cap

Conditionally edible. Can only be consumed when it is fresh, before it turns black. Must be boiled. It mainly grows in large groups on manured areas, in gardens, orchards, fields, near barns, stables, compost heaps, around stumps and rotting tree trunks. Bears fruit several times a year. Season: May to October.

Medicinal uses: Used to treat alcohol dependence. Has strong antibacterial, antiviral and anti-inflammatory (abscesses, furunculosis) effects, treats respiratory diseases (inflammation, bronchitis, SARS, influenza, etc.) and burns. It treats malignant dermatitis, ulcers, other skin diseases. It normalizes the digestive system. It strengthens the immune system, activates anti-tumor protective systems of the body. Used for the prevention and treatment of malignant tumors and benign formations.

33

Coprinus comatus - Shaggy Ink Cap

Conditionally edible. As food, it can only be consumed when young, before it turns black and after boiling. In some countries it is considered a delicacy (France, Finland, Czech Republic). It grows in groups in unexpected places: on green lawns in cities, in gardens, orchards, and also in pastures, fields, and meadows. Season: June to November.

Medicinal uses: Has strong antibacterial and antifungal effects (aspergillosis, otomycosis), treats diseases caused by Staphylococcus aureus (acne, impetigo, boils, cellulitis, carbuncles, staphylococcal scalded skin syndrome, abscess, pneumonia, meningitis, osteomyelitis, endocarditis, toxic shock, sepsis), abscesses, purulent wounds, enteritis, cystitis and candidiasis (thrush). It has a suppressing effect on hay bacillus. It treats diabetes mellitus. It can be used to normalize the digestive system, to lower cholesterol, for the treatment and prevention of cardiovascular diseases, hemorrhoids. It treats intestinal, paroxysmal and septic escherichiosis. It has an antioxidant effect. The fungus is used for treatment of alcohol dependence in varying degrees.

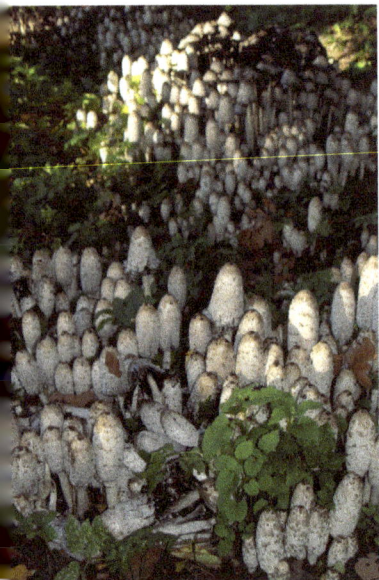

Cortinarius armillatus - Red Banded Webcap

Edible. Grows in small groups or solitary in deciduous and mixed forests, forming mycorrhiza with birch trees. Season: August to October.

Medicinal uses: Has antibacterial and anti-inflammatory (abscesses, furunculosis) effects. Strengthens the immune system, activates anti-tumor protective systems of the body. Used for the prevention and treatment of malignant tumors and benign formations.

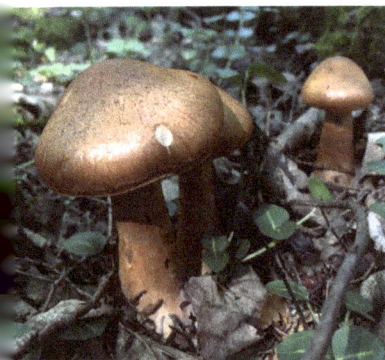

34

Cordyceps militaris - Scarlet Caterpillarclub

Edible. It parasitizes on butterflies (caterpillars), ants, and flies. The mushroom prefers pine and small-leaved forests with an abundance of dead wood and well-developed shrubs (raspberry, mountain ash) and plants (nettle). It grows in gardens, meadows, and mixed forests. Season: June to October.

Medicinal uses: Has strong antibacterial and anti-inflammatory effects, treats community-acquired pneumonia, pulmonary tuberculosis, sinusitis, otitis media, respiratory diseases, bronchial asthma. It has antioxidant and antitoxic effects, treats diseases of the circulatory system, diabetes mellitus, liver and kidney diseases. It is used in gerontology, as it is said to slow down the aging process. It has a tonic effect and rejuvenating properties, is used to lower cholesterol and to prevent atherosclerosis. It has an adaptogenic effect under stress, treats impotence and is used as an aphrodisiac. It treats obesity and cellulite, to enhance hematopoiesis. It has sedative and calming effects. The fungus can be used for the treatment of intestinal, paroxysmal and septic escherichiosis and food poisoning (including vomiting and diarrhea symptoms), and cryptococcosis. It has a suppressing effect on hay bacillus.

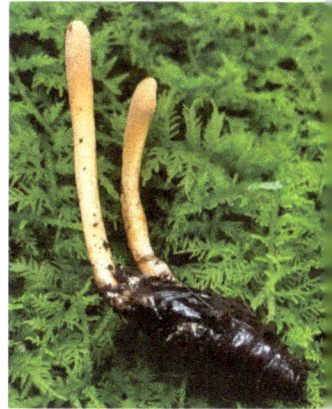

Cortinarius collinitus - Belted Slimy Cort

Edible. Grows in small groups or solitary in deciduous and coniferous forests. It forms mycorrhiza with both birch and, possibly, with pine. The fungus can be found in wet places, along the edges of swamps, on bumps, in mosses. Season: August to October.

Medicinal uses: Has strong antibacterial and anti-inflammatory effects. Used for the prevention and treatment of hypertension. It lowers the level of cholesterol in the blood. It strengthens the immune system and activates anti-tumor protective systems of the body. Used for the prevention and treatment of malignant tumors and benign formations.

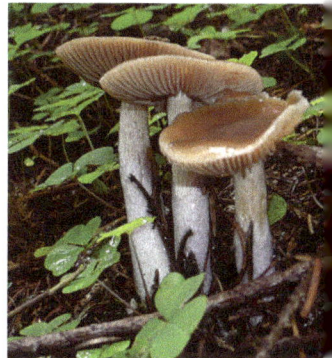

Craterellus cornucopioides - Horn of Plenty

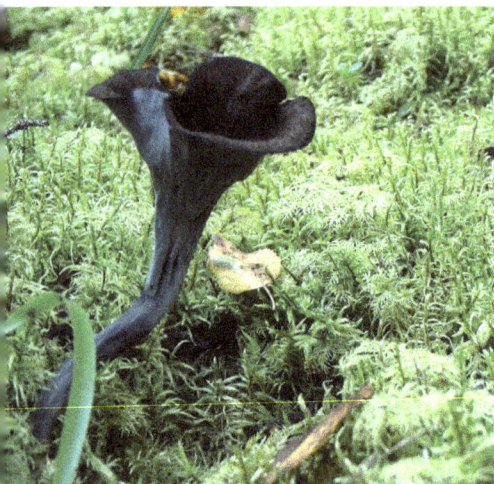

Edible. Considered a delicacy fungus. It grows in moist deciduous and mixed forests, either solitary or in multiple groups, in the grass, in the moss, on roadsides and paths, at the edges of ditches, in open places. It is found in mountainous areas too. Season: July to November.

Medicinal uses: Has an anti-mutagenic effect. Can be used for the prevention and treatment of Alzheimer's disease and senile dementia. It strengthens the immune system and activates anti-tumor protective systems of the body. Used for the prevention and treatment of malignant tumors and benign formations.

Crepidotus mollis - Soft Slipper

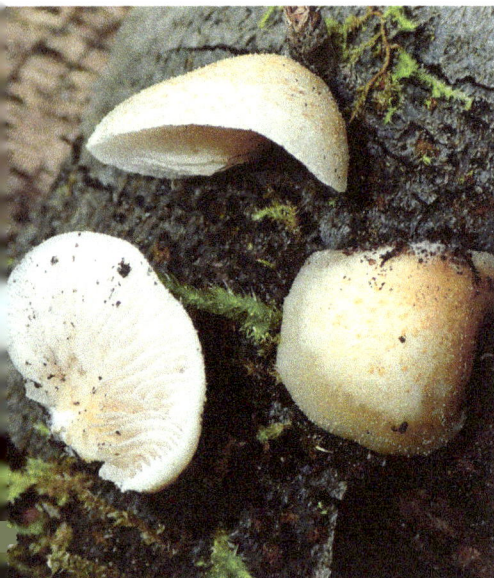

Edible. Grows in large groups or solitary, on decaying, dead or dry wood of many species of trees in deciduous and mixed forests, causing white rot. Sometimes found in hollows of living trees, and on processed wood. It prefers to grow on hardwood, including maple, poplar, alder, beech, oak, sycamore and others. Season: May to October.

Medicinal uses: Strengthens the immune system, used to activate anti-tumor protective systems of the body, and for the prevention and treatment of malignant tumors and benign formations.

36

Cryptoporus volvatus - Cryptic Globe Fungus

Inedible. Fruit bodies are like flattened balls from below, with a rudimentary lateral pedicle. It grows in groups or solitary on the trunks of conifers that were damaged by insects, fire, or other things. Relic species, frequently seen in cedar and broad-leaved forests, causes grey-brown rot. Season: all year round.

Medicinal uses: Has antibacterial and anti-inflammatory effects, treats diseases of the respiratory system (inflammation, bronchitis, acute respiratory viral infection, influenza, asthma). It provides an immuno-stimulating and immuno-modulating action. Can be used for the

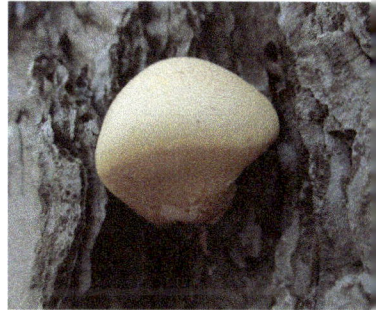

treatment of brain diseases (multiple sclerosis, chorea, epilepsy, vasospasm) and treats joint diseases (arthrosis, arthritis, rheumatism, polyarthritis, osteochondrosis, psoriatic arthritis). It treats allergies and diseases of the circulatory system and improves hematopoiesis. Used in gerontology, as it is said to slow down the aging process. It normalizes fat metabolism and treats obesity and cellulite.

Daedaleopsis confragosa - Thin Walled Maze Polypore

Inedible. Fruit bodies are annual, less often perennial, sessile, semisolid, single, or grow one above the other. This is a parasite that grows on the trunks of hardwood (oak, beech, birch, willow, etc.), on stumps, and on damaged or dead trees, causing white rot. A healing tea is prepared from the fungus. Season: all year round.

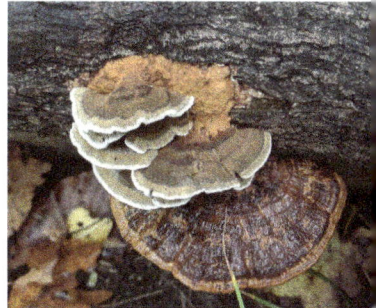

Medicinal uses: Has antibacterial, antifungal and antioxidant effects, treats diseases caused by Staphylococcus aureus (acne, impetigo, boils, abscesses, carbuncles, staphylococcal scalded skin syndrome, pneumonia, meningitis, osteomyelitis, endocarditis, toxic shock, sepsis) and septic wounds. It has a suppressing effect on hay bacillus. Can be used to treat food poisoning, infection of the kidneys and urinary tract, enteritis and cystitis. It treats hypertension, intestinal, paroxysmal and septic escherichiosis, microsporia.

Fistulina hepatica - Beefsteak Fungus

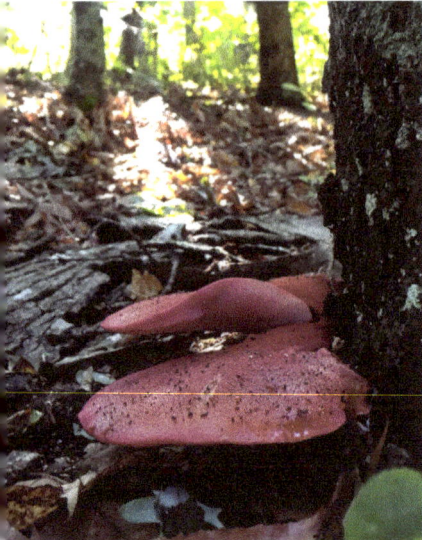

Edible at a young age. It grows in forests and parks on the dying trunks of oaks, chestnuts, eucalyptus and other hardwood trees. Season: August to October.

Medicinal uses: Has strong antibacterial and antioxidant effects, treats typhoid, paratyphoid fever. It has an anti-hilmintic effect (enterobiosis, taeniasis, trichuriasis, ascariasis, hookworm, giardiasis, schistosomiasis, clonorchiasis), treats intestinal, paroxysmal and septic escherichiosis. It has a suppressing effect on hay bacillus. It can be used for the treatment of gout and gouty arthritis.

Flammulina velutipes - Winter Mushroom

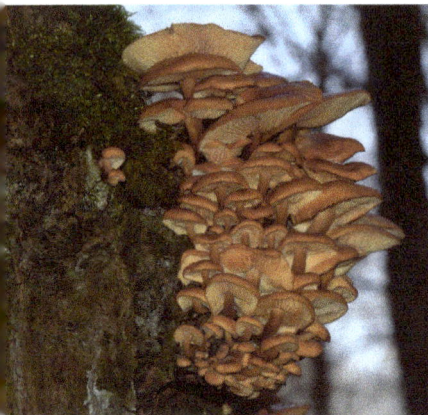

Edible. Grows in mixed forests in large groups on living and dead trees (willow, poplar). Can be found on stumps, trunks, roots, in gardens, parks, on the banks of streams. Fructifies during winter thaws, sometimes it can be found under snow. Season: September to March.

Medicinal uses: Has antibacterial, antiviral and anti-inflammatory effects, treats diseases caused by Staphylococcus aureus. The mushroom can be used to treat diseases of the brain (sclerosis, chorea, epilepsy, vasospasms), Alzheimer's disease, senile dementia. It used in gerontology, as it is said to slow down the aging process, and as a cosmetic agent. It normalizes the digestion system and treats liver diseases. It has a mild laxative effect. It can be used to treat cardiovascular diseases. It treats food poisoning, intestinal, paroxysmal and septic escherichiosis. It has anti-anoxic effects. It normalizes the metabolism and is used as restorative remedy.

38

Fomes applanatus - Artist's Bracket

Inedible. Fruit body is perennial, of various sizes, flat, sessile, rarely hooflike. It grows everywhere on stumps and weakened trunks of deciduous (birch, aspen, willow, oak) and occasionally on coniferous (fir, pine, larch, spruce) trees. The fungus rarely grows on living trees (oak, poplar), causes white or yellowish-white rot of wood and roots. A healing tea is prepared from the fungus. Season: all year round.

Medicinal uses: Has antibacterial and anti-inflammatory effects, treats diseases caused by Staphylococcus aureus (acne, impetigo, boils, cellulitis, carbuncles, staphylococcal scalded skin syndrome, abscess, pneumonia, meningitis, osteomyelitis, endocarditis, toxic shock, sepsis) and diseases of the respiratory system. It has analgesic and antipyretic effects. Can be used for the treatment of tuberculosis and to treat intestinal, paroxysmal and septic escherichiosis. It exerts a tonic effect.

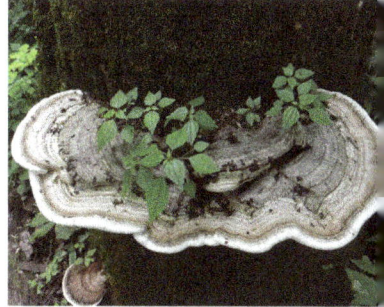

Fomes fomentarius - Tinder Fungus

Inedible. Fruit body is perennial, sessile, hooflike. It parasitizes and grows on the trunks of hardwood (oak, beech, birch, aspen, alder), on stumps, and on weakened and dead trees. A healing tea is prepared from the fungus. Season: all year round.

Medicinal uses: Has antibacterial and antiviral effects, treats diseases of the respiratory system (inflammation, bronchitis, acute respiratory viral infection, influenza, asthma), pneumonia, abscesses, purulent wounds, enteritis and cystitis. It has a suppressing effect on hay bacillus. Can be used for the treatment of diseases of the nervous system and joint diseases (arthrosis, arthritis, rheumatism, polyarthritis, osteochondrosis, psoriatic arthritis), treats ingrown nails. Normalizes the digestive system and treats gastrointestinal diseases. Has a hemostatic effect (on wounds). Lowers cholesterol and is used as mild laxative agent. It has a sedative effect and normalizes the body metabolism. Used as a restorative and tonic remedy.

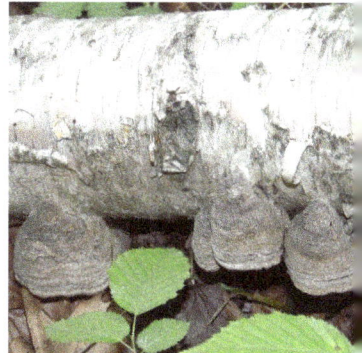

39

Fomes nigricans - Willow Bracket

Inedible. Fruit bodies are perennial. Parasitizes and grows on the trunks of deciduous trees and on stumps of damaged and dead trees, mainly on willows and birches, less often on alders, hornbeam, beech, oaks, chestnuts. A healing tea is prepared from the fungus. Season: all year round.

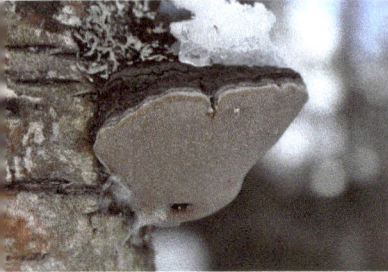

Medicinal uses: Enhances the immune system, activates anti-tumor protective systems of the body. Used for the prevention and treatment of malignant tumors and benign formations.

Fomitopsis officinalis - Quinine Conk

Inedible. Grows and parasitizes on the trunks of old conifererous trees (Douglas firs, Siberian cedars, spruce, larch, etc.) A healing tea is prepared from the fungus. Season: all year round.

Medicinal uses: Has strong antibacterial and antiviral effects, suppresses the activity of influenza viruses and HIV, treats respiratory diseases (inflammation, bronchitis, acute respiratory viral infection, influenza, etc.). It normalizes the digestive system and treats gastrointestinal diseases, diabetes mellitus, pleurisy, pancreatitis, dysbiosis, restores liver function and is used for the treatment of liver cirrhosis and hepatitis. It can be used for the treatment of diseases of the nervous system and endocrine gland diseases. It treats pulmonary tuberculosis and pseudotuberculosis, pneumonia and chronic bronchitis. It can be used as a sleeping pill and as a sedative. It effectively reduces sweating and treats sarcoidosis. It can be used for treatment of constipation and has a mild laxative effect. It normalizes body metabolism, treats obesity and cellulite. Used as a restorative agent. It has an antitoxic effect and is used as the main component of the antidote to all known poisons. Removes carcinogens from the body.

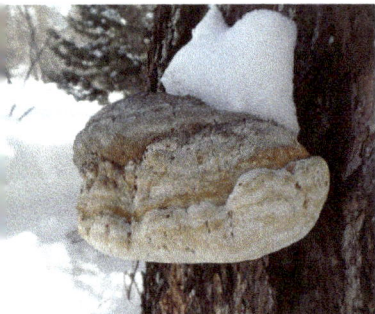

Fomitopsis pinicola - Red Banded Polypore

Inedible. Fruit bodies of the fungus are perennial, sessile, adhering sideways. Parasitizes and grows on the trunks of old deciduous and coniferous trees (tree stumps, fallen trees, dead wood). The fruiting bodies can be found on alive but weakened trees at the bottom of the trunk. A healing tea is prepared from the fungus. Season: all year round.

Medicinal uses: Has antibacterial and anti-inflammatory effects, treats diseases caused by Staphylococcus aureus (acne, impetigo, furunculus, phlegmon, carbuncles, staphylococcal burn-like skin syndrome, abscess, pneumonia, meningitis, osteomyelitis, endocarditis, sepsis, infectious-toxic shock). It can be used for the prevention and treatment of gastrointestinal diseases, foodborne toxic infections, including vomiting and diarrhea symptoms, for the treatment of intestinal, paroxysmal and septic escherichiosis. It exerts a tonic effect, has immuno-stimulating and immuno-modulating action.

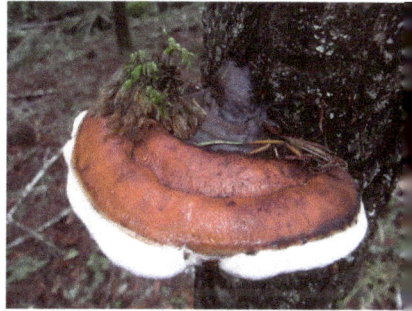

Ganoderma brownii - Artist's Conk

Inedible. This perennial fungus is a concentrically zonate, sessile polypore, its color varies from brown to gray. It grows on the forest litter or live deciduous trees, giving preference to the oak, lime and poplar, causes white rot. A healing tea is prepared from the fungus. Season: all year round.

Medicinal uses: Has strong antibacterial, antiviral and anti-inflammatory effects, treats diseases caused by Staphylococcus aureus (acne, impetigo, boils, cellulitis, carbuncles, staphylococcal scalded skin syndrome, abscess, pneumonia, meningitis, osteomyelitis, endocarditis, toxic shock, sepsis) and respiratory diseases (inflammation, bronchitis, acute respiratory viral infection, influenza, etc.). It can be used for the treatment of pulmonary tuberculosis. It treats intestinal, paroxysmal and septic escherichiosis. It exerts a tonic effect.

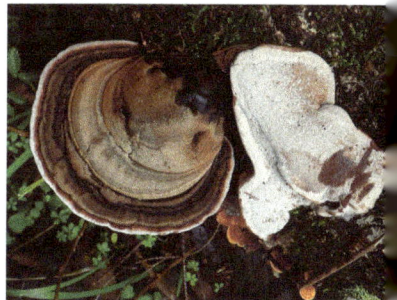

Edible when young. Unique in its chemical composition of useful nutrients. Grows on trunks of eastern hemlock, weak and dying conifers, wood residues, stumps, roots and very rarely on deciduous trees (maple). Season: all year round.

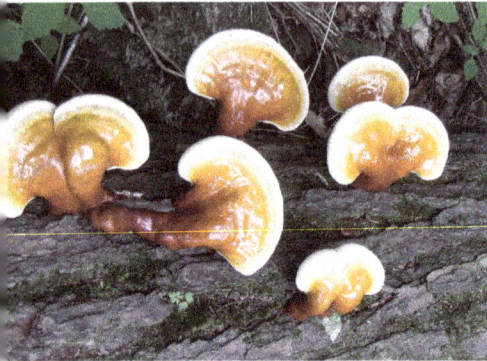

Medicinal uses: Has strong antibacterial and antiviral effects, treats diseases caused by Staphylococcus aureus (acne, impetigo, boils, cellulitis, carbuncles, staphylococcal scalded skin syndrome, abscess, pneumonia, meningitis, osteomyelitis, endocarditis, toxic shock, sepsis). Used to treat diseases of the respiratory system. It treats urethritis, trichomoniasis, ureaplasmosis, meningitis, otitis media, sinusitis, cytomegalovirus, viral-hepatitis, chlamydia, diseases caused by human herpes virus types 1 and 2 (HSV-1 and HSV-2) and by influenza viruses. Can be used to treat diseases of the brain (sclerosis, chorea, epilepsy, vasospasm), Parkinson's disease, Alzheimer's disease, senile dementia, mental illnesses, neuroses. Has an analgesic effect, treats headaches and migraines, muscle pain, cramps, pain in the tendons, numbness of the limbs, lumbago, treats joint diseases (arthrosis, arthritis, rheumatism, polyarthritis, osteochondrosis, psoriatic arthritis). Normalizes the digestive system and is used to treat liver and kidney diseases. Pro-

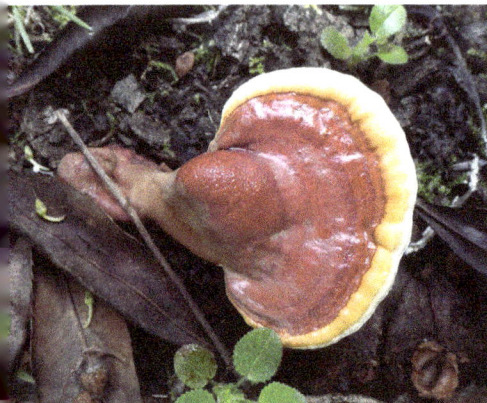

vides an immuno-stimulating and immuno-modulating action. The mushroom is used in gerontology, as it is believed to slow down the aging process. It treats cardiovascular diseases, thrombosis, hypertension. Has antioxidant effects and provides antitoxic action. Normalizes the metabolism and treats obesity and cellulite. Can be used to treat eye diseases and improve hearing. It has an adaptogenic effect under stress. Used as a restorative and as a tonic remedy.

Ganoderma oregonense - Western Varnish Shelf

Inedible. The color of the fungus varies from bright purple to reddish-brown. It has a unique chemical composition of useful nutrients. Grows solitary or in groups in coniferous forests on weakened and dying trees, on decaying trunks, stumps, or roots. A healing tea is prepared from the fungus. Season: all year round.

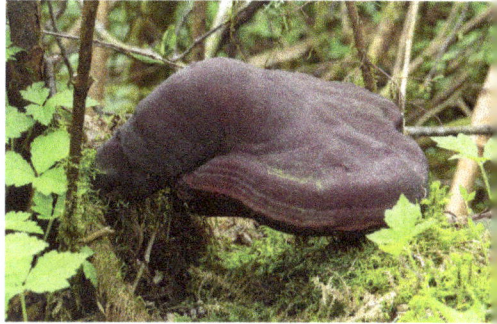

Medicinal uses: Has antibacterial and antiviral effects, treats allergies. It provides an immuno-stimulating and immuno-modulating action. It has antioxidant and hepato-protective effects.

Ganoderma sinense - Black Ganoderma

Inedible. Has a unique chemical composition of useful nutrients. Grows solitary in coniferous forests on weak and dying coniferous trees, woody debris, tree trunks, stumps, roots. A healing tea or wine are prepared from the fungus. Season: all year round.

Medicinal uses: Has antibacterial and antiviral effects, treats diseases caused by Staphylococcus aureus (acne, impetigo, boils, cellulitis, carbuncles, staphylococcal scalded skin syndrome, abscess, pneumonia, meningitis, osteomyelitis, endocarditis, toxic shock, sepsis). It normalizes the digestive system and treats liver and kidney diseases. It can be used for the treatment of mental illnesses, neuroses. It normalizes the metabolism and treats obesity and cellulite. Has an analgesic effect, treats headaches and migraines, muscle pain, cramps, pain in the tendons, numbness of the limbs, lumbago. It is used in gerontology, as it is said to

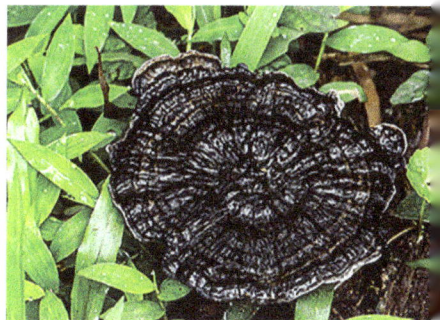

slow down the aging process. Provides an immuno-stimulating and immuno-modulating action. Has antioxidant effects and provides antitoxic action. Strengthens overall condition of the body.

Ganoderma tsugae - Hemlock Varnish Shelf

Inedible. Has a unique chemical composition of useful nutrients. Grows parasitizes, solitary or in groups, on the trunks of eastern hemlock, spruce, weak and dying conifers, on wood residues, on stumps, roots. A healing tea and wine are prepared from the fungus. Season: May to November.

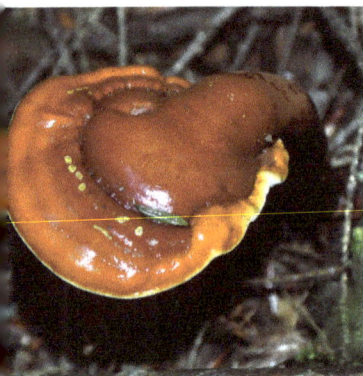

Medicinal uses: Has antibacterial and antiviral effects, treats chronic tracheitis, chronic hepatitis, rheumatoid arthritis. Promotes wound healing. Regulates fat metabolism, treats obesity and cellulite. The mushroom can be used for the prevention and treatment of cardiovascular diseases and cardiopathy, reduces high blood cholesterol and stimulates blood circulation. It treats neurasthenia. Long-term use of the fungus contributes to longevity.

Grifola frondosa - Hen-of-the-Woods

Edible. Grows and parasitizes solitarily or in groups in deciduous forests at the base of weakened and old birch, oak, beech, chestnut trees. Season: August to September.

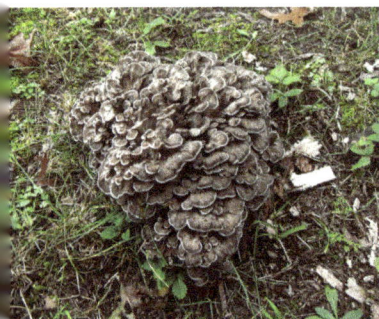

Medicinal uses: Has strong antibacterial, antiviral and anti-inflammatory effects. Can be used to treat poliomyelitis and diseases caused by influenza viruses. Used to treat brain diseases, psoriasis, diabetes mellitus, endocrine gland and joint diseases. It has anti-fungal effects and treats candidiasis (thrush). Can be used to treat hypertension and diseases of the circulatory system, enhances hematopoiesis, lowers cholesterol, treats gastrointestinal and liver diseases. The mushroom normalizes one's metabolism and hormonal level, treats obesity and cellulite. Used as restorative remedy in gerontology. This is not yet a complete list of the medicinal properties of the fungus, which is being supplemented by research.

44

Gyromitra brunnea - Gabled False Morel

Conditionally edible. It needs to be boiled in water for 10 minutes, then drained, after which it may be cooked in many dishes. Grows solitary or in small groups, especially near rotting stumps in beech forests, or in glades. It can also be found in timber clearings, on forest fire clearings, roadsides, near rivulets, in places where ground has been disturbed. Season: March to May.

Medicinal uses: Has antibacterial, antiviral and anti-inflammatory effects, treats diseases of the respiratory system. Has anesthetic effects, treats diseases of the back and joints (arthritis, radiculitis, gout, arthrosis, osteochondrosis, rheumatism, etc.), treats neuralgia, myositis. It can be used for the treatment of eye diseases (cataracts, myopia, glaucoma, farsightedness). It normalizes blood circulation and exerts a tonic effect on the body.

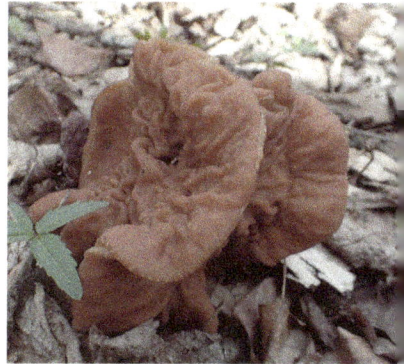

Gyromitra esculenta - False Morel

Conditionally edible. In some countries, considered poisonous. Needs to be boiled in water for 10 minutes, then drained, after which it can be used in cooking. Grows in sandy soils under coniferous trees (pine, spruce) and sometimes in deciduous woodlands (aspen, poplar, birch). It also can be found in timber clearings, on forest fire clearings, along roadsides, near rivulets, or in places where ground has been disturbed. Season: March to June.

Medicinal uses: Has antibacterial, antiviral and anti-inflammatory effects, treats inflammatory processes in the pancreas and improves its function. The mushroom normalizes blood circulation. It used to treat diseases of the respiratory system (bronchitis, acute respiratory viral infection, influenza, etc.). Has anesthetic effects, treats neuralgia, myositis. It can be used for the treatment of eye diseases (cataracts, myopia, glaucoma, farsightedness). The mushroom is used as an appetizer.

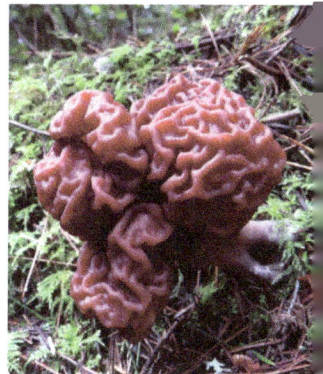

45

Gyromitra gigas - Snow Morel

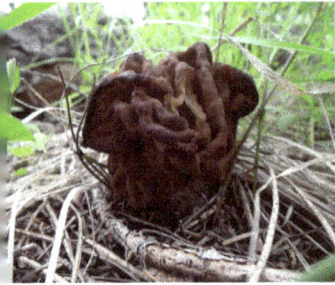

Conditionally edible. Needs to be boiled in water for 10 minutes, then drained, after which it can be used for cooking. It grows in sandy soils in mountain conifer forests, under pine and spruce trees, in deciduous (aspen, poplar, birch) or mixed forests. Season: April to June.

Medicinal uses: Has antibacterial, antiviral and anti-inflammatory effects, treats diseases of the respiratory system, inflammatory processes in the pancreas and improves pancreatic function. Has anesthetic effects, treats neuralgia, myositis, diseases of the back and joints (arthritis, radiculitis, gout, arthrosis, osteochondrosis, rheumatism and others). It can be used to treat eye diseases (cataracts, myopia, glaucoma, farsightedness). It exerts a tonic effect.

Hericium abietis - Bear's Head

Edible. Grows solitary on the trunks of dead or weakened conifer (Douglas fir, hemlock, spruce, cedar pine) trees or on conifer stumps or logs. It occurs in mountainous, less often subarctic conifer forests. Season: August to December.

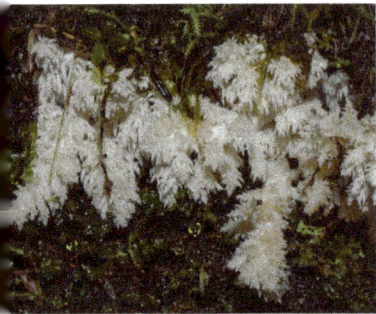

Medicinal uses: Has antibacterial and antiviral effects, treats diseases caused by the bacterium Helicobacter pylori and Staphylococcus aureus, and respiratory diseases. It is used to reduce the side effects of chemotherapy and radiotherapy and removes toxins from the body. It normalizes the function of the liver and kidneys, improves hemoglobin levels in the blood. It can be used to treat diseases of the nervous system (mental illnesses, neuroses), Alzheimer's disease, senile dementia, Parkinson's disease. It normalizes the digestion system and treats gastrointestinal diseases. Has anti-fungal action (aspergillosis, otomycosis). It is used in gerontology, as it is thought to slow down the aging process. It normalizes fat metabolism and treats obesity and cellulite. The mushroom treats impotence, can increase sexual desire and improves the overall health.

46

Hericium americanum - Bear's Head Tooth Fungus

Edible. Grows solitary or in clusters in deciduous, mixed and rarely in coniferous forests on stumps, hardwood logs (ash, beech, oak) or trunks of various types of weakened and living trees. Season: August to November.

Medicinal uses: Used to reduce the side effects of chemotherapy and radiotherapy, and removes toxins from the body. Has strong antibacterial and antiviral effects. It normalizes the digestive system, functioning of the liver and kidneys, improves the level of hemoglobin in blood and treats gastrointestinal diseases, obesity and cellulite. It can be used to treat diseases of the nervous system (mental illnesses, neuroses), Alzheimer's disease, senile dementia, Parkinson's disease. The mushroom treats impotence and increases sexual desire. Has antifungal action (aspergillosis, otomycosis). It is used in gerontology and improves overall health and metabolism.

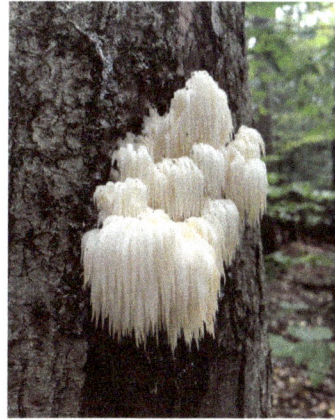

Hericium erinaceus - Lion's Mane Mushroom

Edible. Grows solitary on the trunks of dead or weakened deciduous trees (birch, oak, beech). Season: August to October.

Medicinal uses: Used to reduce side effects of chemotherapy, radiotherapy and to remove toxins from the body. It provides an immuno-stimulating and immuno-modulating action. Has strong antibacterial and antiviral effects. It can be used to treat the nervous system (mental illnesses, neuroses), Alzheimer's disease, senile dementia, Parkinson's disease. It normalizes digestion system, the work of the liver, kidneys, improves the formula of blood and the level of hemoglobin, and for regulation of the blood circulation. It treats gastrointestinal diseases and impotence and can increase sexual desire. Used in gerontology, as it is thought to slow down the aging process. Normalizes metabolism and can be used as restorative remedy and for improvement of overall health.

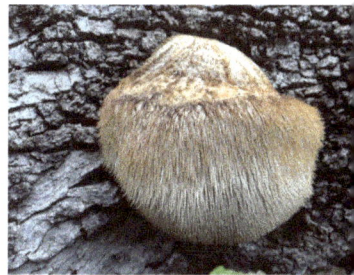

Hydnum repandum - Sweet Tooth

Edible. Considered to be one of the best mushrooms in France. Grows in groups or solitary on fallen leaves, needles, moss cover in mixed and deciduous forests, forming mycorrhiza with different species of trees. Season: July to November.

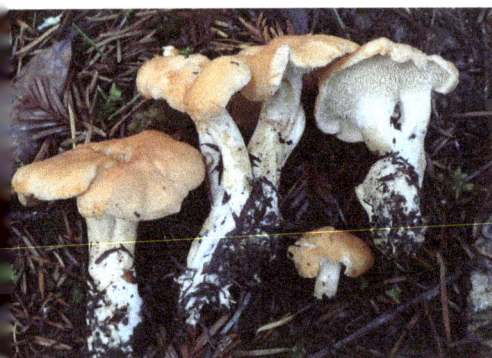

Medicinal uses: Has antibacterial effects, treats diseases caused by Staphylococcus aureus (acne, impetigo, furunculus, phlegmon, carbuncles, staphylococcal burn-like skin syndrome, abscess, pneumonia, meningitis, osteomyelitis, endocarditis, sepsis, infectious-toxic shock), hospital-acquired infections. The mushroom lowers cholesterol in the blood.

Hypholoma lateritium - Brick Cap

Conditionally edible. In North America and Japan the mushroom is considered edible. It must be boiled in water for 10 minutes, then drained before being used in dishes. Grows in large groups on fallen leaves, in moss, on decaying trunks, on and around stumps, on rotting wood (oak, beech, birch) in deciduous and coniferous forests. Season: July to December.

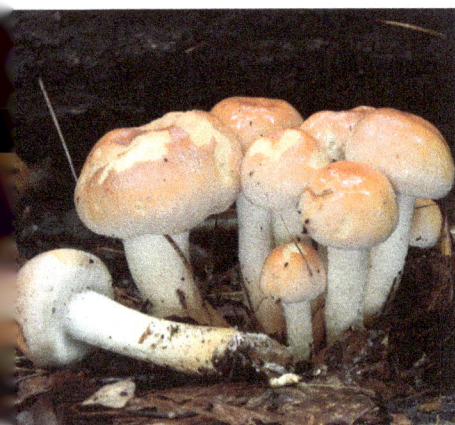

Medicinal uses: Has antioxidant properties, treats periodontitis and joint diseases (arthrosis, arthritis, rheumatism, polyarthritis, osteochondrosis, psoriatic arthritis). It can be used to treat amnesia. It provides an immuno-stimulating and immuno-modulating action. Can be used for the treatment of eye diseases, improves vision. It treats gastrointestinal diseases and is used as an emetic agent. The mushroom normalizes fat metabolism, treats obesity and cellulite.

48

Indian sea rice

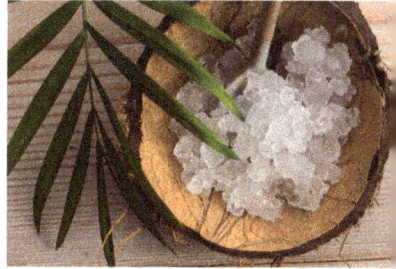

Inedible. Indian sea rice is a symbiotic group of bacteria and microorganisms of the genus Zoogloea and has a mucous formation, similar to ordinary rice. There are two varieties of sea rice: small and large. It is used for preparing a tonic water drink. It can be grown in all countries of the world all year round.

Medicinal uses: Has antioxidant and anti-inflammatory effects, treats diseases of the digestive system and cardiovascular diseases, and prevents development of atherosclerosis. It stimulates metabolic processes and helps to remove toxins from the body, regulates fat metabolism, treats obesity and diseases of the joints. Used to prevent chronic fatigue syndrome, insomnia and depression. Has a tonic effect, slows down the aging process of the body, normalizes vitality level.

Inonotus obliquus - Chaga Mushroom

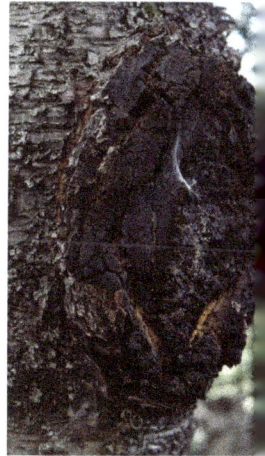

Inedible. Grows on deciduous trees: birch, ash, alder, maple, and elm. It can grow for 10 to 20 years, eventually killing the tree it dwells on. The mushrooms that grow on birch trees have medicinal values. A healing tea is prepared from the fungus. Season: all year round.

Medicinal uses: Has anti-bacterial, antiviral, anti-inflammatory and antifungal effects, treats respiratory diseases, pulmonary tuberculosis, diseases caused by influenza viruses, HIV infection. It can be used to treat diseases of the brain and nervous system. The mushroom contributes to the normal operation of the body's central and peripheral systems. It treats cardiovascular diseases, atherosclerosis and activates hematopoietic functions, normalizes blood pressure and pulse. It treats gastrointestinal disease, liver and kidneys. Has antioxidant, antitoxic and analgesic effects. It treats joint pain, skin diseases (eczema, psoriasis), endocrine gland diseases, diabetes mellitus. It is used in gerontology, as it is thought to slow down the aging process. It treats diseases of the female reproductive system and mastitis. The mushroom improves body energy levels and can be used as restorative remedy.

Kombucha - Tea Fungus

Inedible. In everyday life it is usually called a Tea fungus, which is a symbiosis of acetic acid bacteria and yeast. It is a layered mucous membrane, located on the surface of a liquid nutrient medium (sweet tea or other sweet mixtures). Strains of microorganisms vary depending on the place of origin and produce sweet and sour "tea kvass," slightly aerated. It can be grown in all countries of the world all year round.

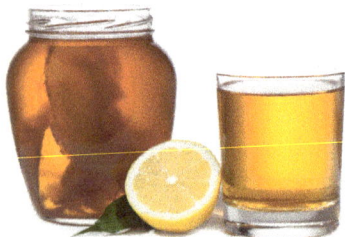

Medicinal uses: Has antibacterial, anti-inflammatory and analgesic effects, improves metabolism. Used for preventing the development of atherosclerosis. Kombucha cleans the blood of toxins. It treats rheumatic heart disease, chronic colds, sore throats. It normalizes the level of glucose in the blood and prevents the consequences of diabetes. It restores and stabilizes the natural microflora in the stomach, used to treat diseases of bladder, stomach, liver, kidneys. Helps regulate blood pressure. Has a calming effect on the nervous system, reduces the symptoms of menopause. It slows down the aging process of the body with regular use, removes pigment spots and warts. Used for getting rid of dandruff and grey hair. Has a tonic effect, eases mental fatigue, normalizes and improves sleep.

Kuehneromyces mutabilis - Sheathed Woodtuft

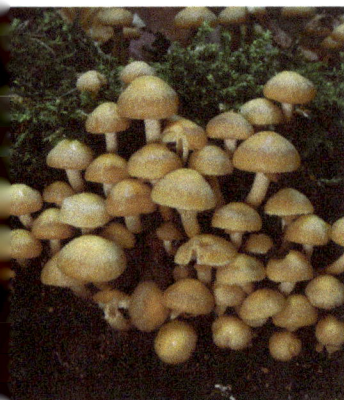

Edible. Grows in dense colonies on dead wood, on decaying wood fragments, on rotting leaves and stumps. It prefers birch, beech, alder and other trees in mixed and deciduous forests. Season: April to November, in mild climates all year round.

Medicinal uses: Has antibacterial and antiviral effects, treats diseases caused by Staphylococcus aureus and by influenza viruses. It can be used for the treatment of endocrine gland diseases, intestinal, paroxysmal and septic escherichiosis.

Edible. It grows solitary or in groups in coniferous and mixed forests, forming mycorrhiza with spruce, pine, and larch trees. Season: from July to October.

Medicinal uses: Enhances the immune system, activates anti-tumor protective systems of the body. Used for prevention and treatment of malignant tumors and benign formations. It has antibacterial effects.

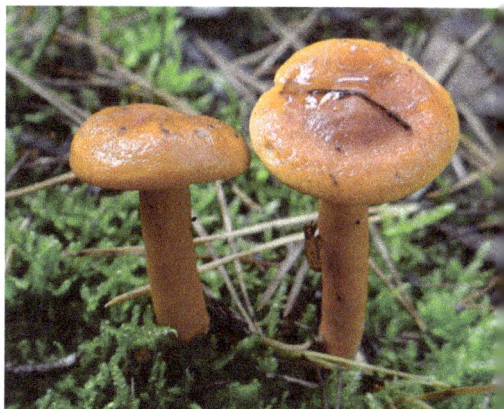

Lactarius deliciosus - Safron Milkcap

Edible. The mushroom grows in groups on sandy soils and forms mycorrhiza with pine. Also often seen in pine and spruce plantations, in wind-sheltered forest belts, in grass, among the moss on pine fringes. Season: July to November.

Medicinal uses: Has antibacterial effects, treats diseases caused by bacteria: Escherichia coli, Micrococcus luteus, Staphylococcus aureus, Salmonella thyphi, Klebsiella pneumoniae, Pseudomonas aeruginosa, Corynebacterium xerosis, Bacillus cereus, Bacillus megaterium, Mycobacterium smegmatis, Candida albicans, and Saccharomyces cerevisiae. Treats pulmonary tuberculosis, abscesses,

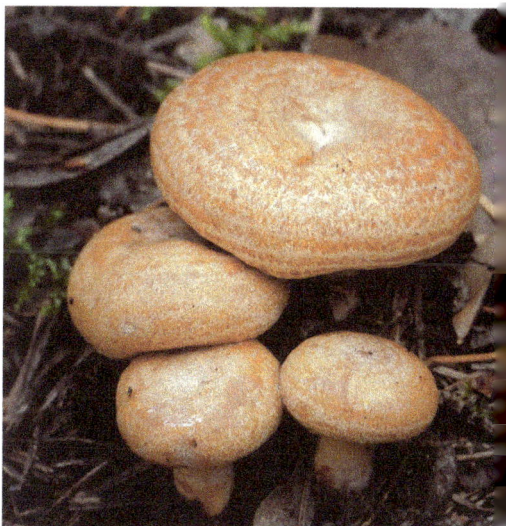

septic wounds, enteritis and cystitis. Has antifungal effects, treats candidiasis (thrush). It removes bad odor from the skin and mucous membranes. It provides an immuno-stimulating and immuno-modulating action, improves vision.

Lactarius deterrimus - False Saffron Milkcap

Edible. Can be found in groups in spruce forests on coniferous litter, on spruce edges, in spruce plantations and mixed forests (birch, oak). It also grows in mountainous areas, in young pine forests, and in parks. Season: June to November.

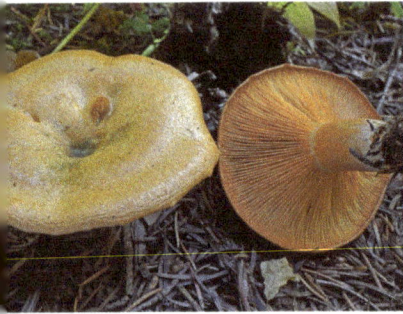

Medicinal uses: Has antibacterial effects, treats diseases caused by bacteria: Escherichia coli, Micrococcus luteus, Staphylococcus aureus, Salmonella thyphi, Klebsiella pneumoniae, Pseudomonas aeruginosa, Corynebacterium xerosis, Bacillus cereus, Bacillus megaterium, Mycobacterium smegmatis, Candida albicans, and Saccharomyces cerevisiae. Has antifungal effects, treats candidiasis (thrush). It can be used for the prevention and treatment of pulmonary tuberculosis, enteritis and cystitis, abscesses, purulent and non-healing wounds, ulcers, rheumatism. Has an antioxidant effect, normalizes the body's metabolism and treats metabolic disorders. It improves vision, provides an immuno-stimulating and immuno-modulating action, and is used as a restorative remedy.

Lactarius flavidulus - Kihatsutake

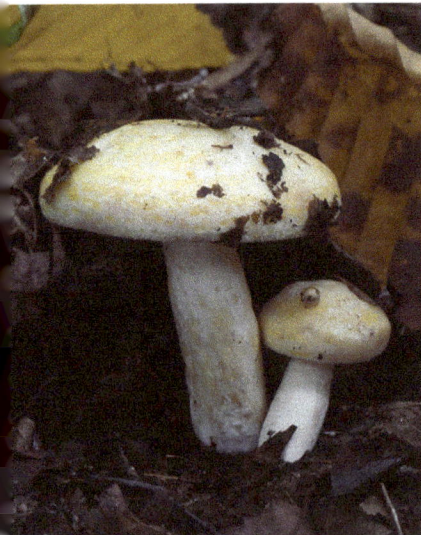

Edible. Can be found in groups in spruce forests on coniferous litter, occurs on spruce edges, in spruce plantations and mixed forests (birch, oak). It also grows in mountainous areas, in young pine forests, and in parks. Season: June to November.

Medicinal uses: Has antibacterial effects, strengthens the immune system, activates anti-tumor protective systems of the body. Used to prevent and treat malignant tumors (sarcoma-180) and benign formations.

Lactarius helvus - Fenugreek Milkcap

Conditionally edible. Must be boiled for 10 minutes in water, then drained, after which it can be used in any dish. The mushroom can be found in coniferous, deciduous and mixed forests, forming mycorrhiza with spruce, pine, and birch trees. It grows solitary or in groups in moist coniferous forests, among the moss, and on the outskirts of sphagnum bogs. Season: July to September.

Medicinal uses: Enhances the immune system, activates anti-tumor protective systems of the body. Used for the prevention and treatment of malignant tumors and benign formations. Has antibacterial effects.

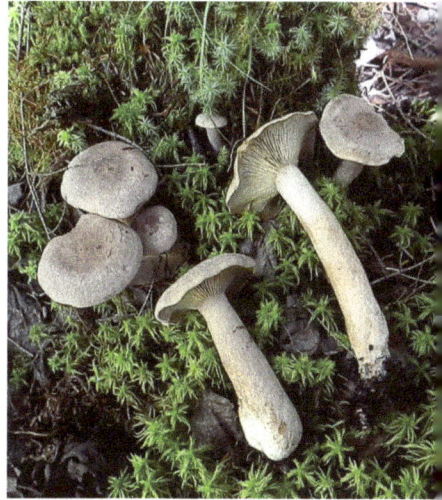

Lactarius piperatus - Peppery Milkcap

Edible. Grows in small groups in the grass in deciduous and mixed forests (birch, oak) and rarely in conifers. The fungus forms mycorrhiza with many deciduous trees, including hazel trees. Season: July to September.

Medicinal uses: Has antibacterial and analgesic effects, treats pulmonary tuberculosis, food poisoning and infections of the kidneys and urinary tract, blenorrhea (acute purulent conjuctivitis). The mushroom helps to remove and dissolve stones in the gallbladder and kidneys. It can be used to treat muscle pain, cramps, pain in the tendons, numbness of the limbs, lumbago. Has an antioxidant effect, treats warts, intestinal, paroxysmal and septic escherichiosis. It normalizes the body's metabolism and treats metabolic disorders.

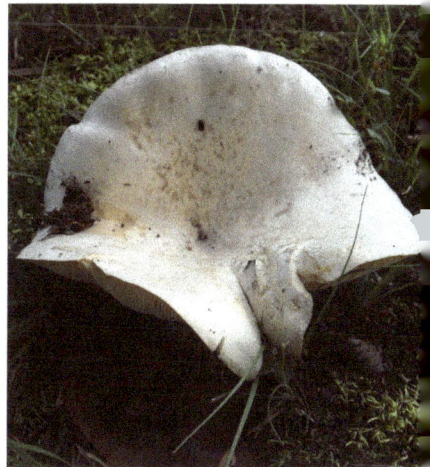

53

Lactarius salmonicolor - Milky Agaric

Edible. It grows on sandy soils in wind-sheltered forest belts, in the grass, among mosses, and on fringes of fir trees. Season: July to November.

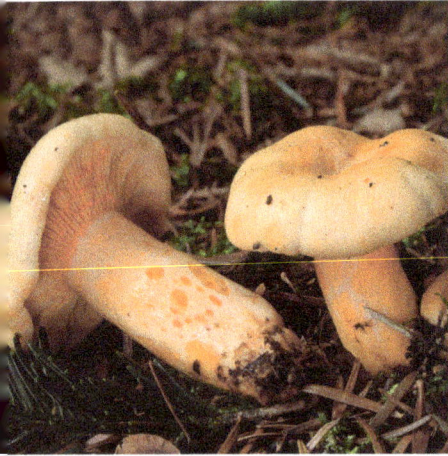

Medicinal uses: Has strong antibacterial effects, treats diseases caused by bacteria: Escherichia coli, Micrococcus luteus, Staphylococcus aureus, Salmonella thyphi, Klebsiella pneumoniae, Pseudomonas aeruginosa, Corynebacterium xerosis, Bacillus cereus, Bacillus megaterium, Mycobacterium smegmatis, Candida albicans, and Saccharomyces cerevisiae. Used to treat tuberculosis, rheumatism. The mushroom normalizes metabolism and treats metabolic disorders. Has antioxidant effects and improves vision.

Lactarius sanguifluus - Bloody Milkcap

Edible. Grows on sandy soils in pine plantations, in wind-sheltered forest belts, in the grass, among the moss, and on pine forest edges. Season: July to November.

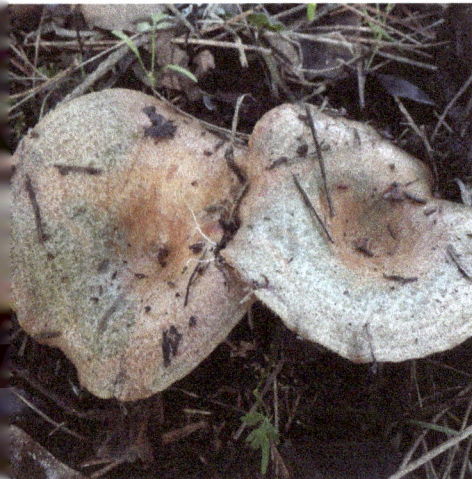

Medicinal uses: Has strong antibacterial effects, treats diseases caused by bacteria: Escherichia coli, Micrococcus luteus, Staphylococcus aureus, Salmonella thyphi, Klebsiella pneumoniae, Pseudomonas aeruginosa, Corynebacterium xerosis, Bacillus cereus, Bacillus megaterium, Mycobacterium smegmatis, Candida albicans, and Saccharomyces cerevisiae. Treats tuberculosis and rheumatism. Normalizes metabolism and treats metabolic disorders. The mushroom improves vision.

Lactarius vellereus - Fleecy Milkcap

Conditionally edible. Must be boiled in water for 10 minutes, then drained, after which it can be cooked in any dish. Grows in small groups among the grass or moss in deciduous and mixed forests (birch, aspen, oak), forming mycorrhiza with many species of trees. Season: July to September.

Medicinal uses: Has antibacterial, analgesic and anti-inflammatory effects (abscesses, furunculosis). It can be used to treat muscle pain, cramps, pain in the tendons, numbness of the limbs, lumbago. It normalizes the body's metabolism and can be used as restorative remedy.

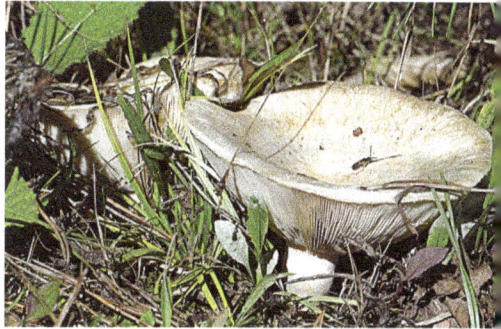

Lactarius volemus - Weeping Milkcap

Edible. Grows in small groups or solitary among the grass of deciduous and mixed forests (commonly birch), forming mycorrhiza with many species of trees. It is a rare fungus. It prefers damp places, but can also be found in the mountains at an altitude of 1000m above sea level. Season: August to October.

Medicinal uses: Has antibacterial and anti-inflammatory effects (abscesses, furunculosis). It treats joint diseases (arthrosis, arthritis, rheumatism, polyarthritis, osteochondrosis, psoriatic arthritis). The mushrooms normalize metabolism, remove toxins from the body and help to cope with obesity. With their regular use, the work of the nervous system is normalized, neuroses and depressions pass. It is used to treat pulmonary emphysema, gallstone disease and urolithiasis. It can be used to strengthen the mucous membranes of the lungs and bronchi, and to treat tuberculosis.

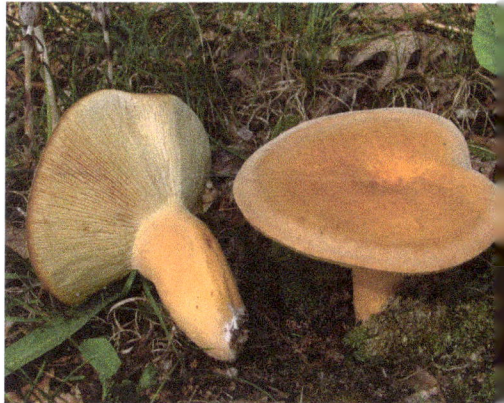

55

Laetiporus sulphureus - Chicken of the Woods

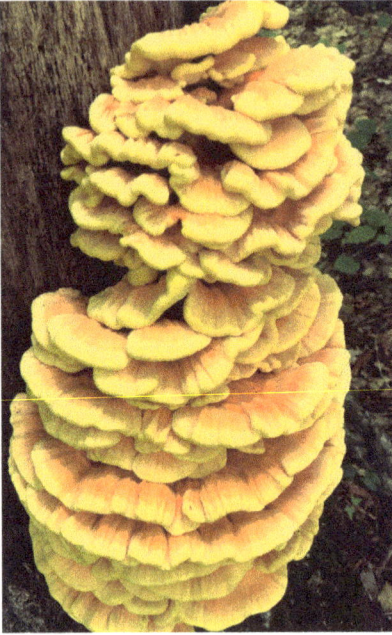

Edible. Grows parasitically, solitarily or in groups, on the trunks of weakened or dead birch, fruit trees, willow, linden, birch, poplar, oak, cedar, walnut, chestnut, maple, pine, larch, spruce and other trees. Season: May to October.

Medicinal uses: Has antibacterial and antiviral effects, treats diseases caused by HIV, respiratory diseases, malaria. It can be used for prevention and treatment of diabetes mellitus and thrombosis. It treats liver diseases, bile duct diseases and intestinal, paroxysmal and septic escherichiosis. Has a laxative effect.

Lentinellus cochleatus - Aniseed Cockleshell

Edible when young. It grows in deciduous forests in large groups near the base of young and dead maple trees, on or near wood of rotten stumps (oak), dead tree trunks, on woody residue. The mushroom emits a pungent smell of anise. Season: June to November.

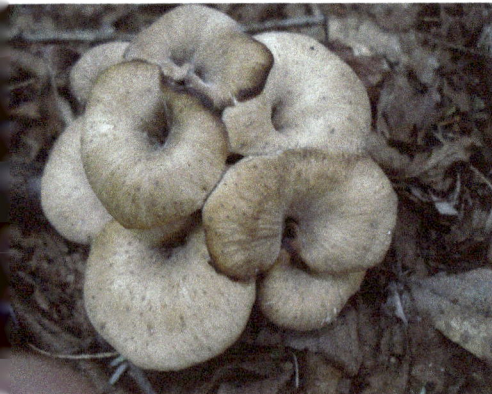

Medicinal uses: Has antibacterial and antiviral effects, suppresses the activity of influenza and HIV viruses, treats intestinal, paroxysmal and septic escherichiosis. Has antifungal effects, treats candidiasis (thrush). Has a suppressing effect on hay bacillus. It provides an immuno-stimulating and immuno-modulating action.

56

Lentinus velutinus - Panus Velutinus

Edible when young. It grows in small groups on decaying wood, on stumps, on dead tree trunks in deciduous and coniferous forests. Season: June to September.

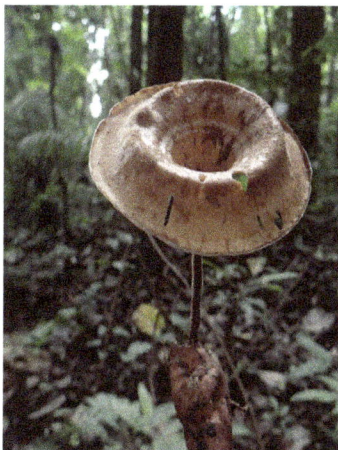

Medicinal uses: Has antiviral effects, suppresses the activity of influenza viruses and HIV. It enhances the immune system, activates anti-tumor protective systems of the body, and is used for the prevention and treatment of malignant tumors and benign formations.

Lenzites betulina - Gilled Polypore

Inedible. Grows in large groups on decaying wood, on the stumps and trunks of dead trees, as well as on dry wood debris of various tree species in deciduous and coniferous forests. The mushroom causes white rot of wood, often destroying the foundations of untreated wooden houses. A healing tea is prepared from the fungus. Season: July to November.

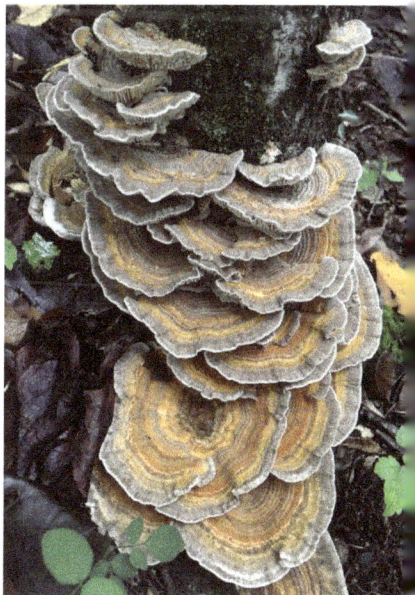

Medicinal uses: Has antibacterial and antiviral effects, treats diseases of the respiratory system (inflammation, bronchitis, acute respiratory viral infection, influenza, etc.), treats hospital-acquired infections, abscesses, septic wounds, enteritis and cystitis, HIV infection. Has a suppressing effect on hay bacillus. Has antioxidant effects, treats muscle pain, cramps, pain in the tendons, numbness of the limbs, lumbago. Has anti-fungal effects, treats candidiasis (thrush). It can be used for the treatment of intestinal, paroxysmal and septic escherichiosis, salmonellosis.

57

Lepiota aspera - Freckled Dapperling

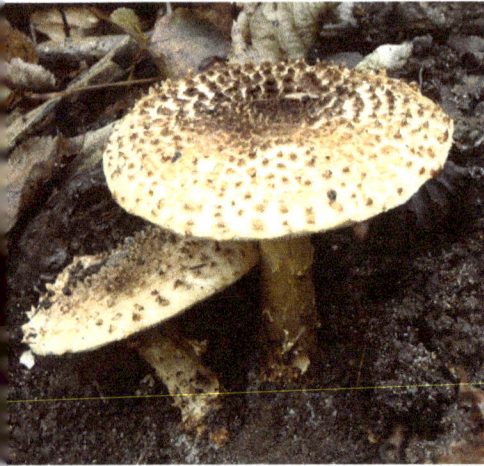

Inedible. Not compatible with alcohol. It grows in groups or solitary on decaying wood in wet deciduous and mixed forests, near roads, on lawns, in parks, gardens, rotted debris, or on wood shavings. Season: August to October.

Medicinal uses: Has antibacterial effects and suppresses hay bacillus. It can be used for the treatment of intestinal, paroxysmal and septic escherichiosis. The mushroom is used to treat alcohol dependence in varying degrees.

Lepista nuda - Clitocybe Nuda

Edible. Grows solitary or in groups on decomposing leaves, on fallen pine needles, around piles of straw, firewood, compost heaps, and wood shavings in mixed (spruce, oak) and coniferous (spruce, pine) forests, sometimes forming "fairy rings". Season: September to October, and in warm places from September to December (up to the first frost).

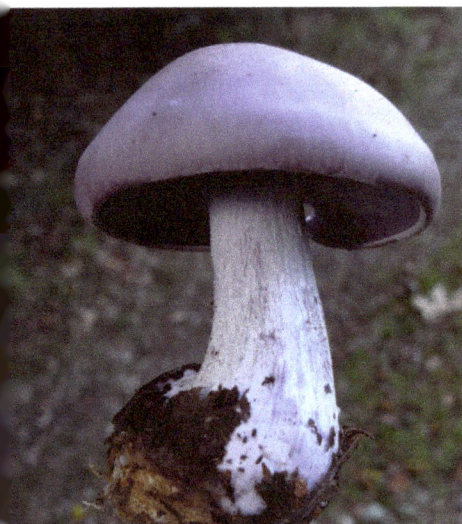

Medicinal uses: Has antibacterial effects, treats diseases caused by Staphylococcus aureus (acne, impetigo, boils, cellulitis, carbuncles, staphylococcal scalded skin syndrome, abscess, pneumonia, meningitis, osteomyelitis, endocarditis, toxic shock, sepsis), treats intestinal, paroxysmal and septic escherichiosis. It can be used for the treatment of acute glomerulonephritis, rheumatism and angina. Treats diabetes mellitus. Has antifungal effects and treats candidiasis (thrush). It can be used for the treatment of diseases of the nervous system.

58

Leucopaxillus gentianeus - Bitter False Funnelcap

Conditionally edible. Must be boiled for 10 minutes in water, then drained, after which it can be cooked in any dish. Grows in groups or solitary on decaying fallen needles and around the trunks of coniferous trees. Season: July to September.

Medicinal uses: Has strong antibacterial effects, treats pulmonary tuberculosis and food poisoning (including vomiting and diarrhea symptoms). It strengthens the immune system, activates the anti-tumor protective systems of the body. Has antioxidant effects. It can be used for the treatment of epilepsy.

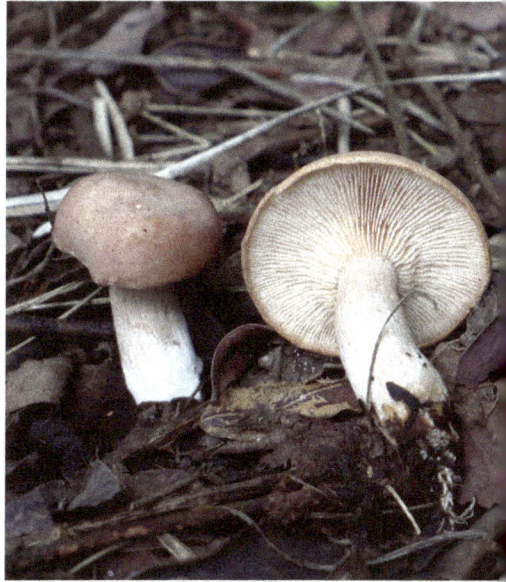

Leucopaxillus giganteus - Giant Funnel

Edible. Grows solitary or in groups, sometimes forming "fairy rings" in pastures, forest clearings, along roads, and in meadows. Season: July to October.

Medicinal uses: Has antibacterial and antioxidant effects, treats diseases caused by Staphylococcus aureus (acne, impetigo, boils, cellulitis, carbuncles, staphylococcal scalded skin syndrome, abscess, pneumonia, meningitis, osteomyelitis, endocarditis, toxic shock, sepsis). Treats typhoid, paratyphoid, tuberculosis of the skin and bones, brucellosis. Has a suppressing effect on hay bacillus. It can be used for the treatment of epilepsy.

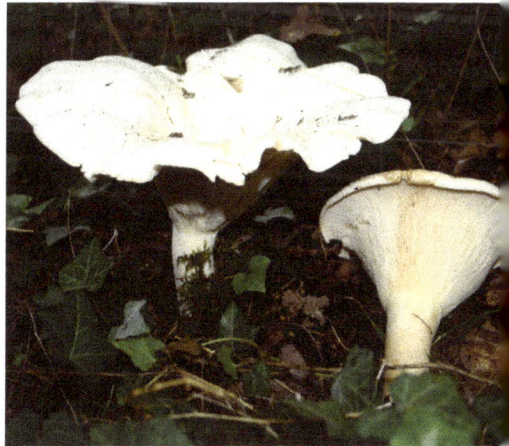

Lycoperdon excipuliforme - Long-Stemmed Puffball

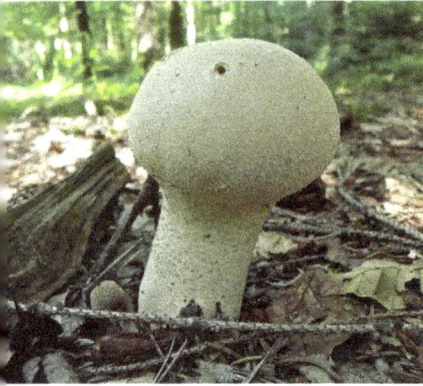

Edible when young, while the flesh is firm, elastic, and white. It grows in groups or solitary on pastures, clearings, forest edges, open fertilized ground. Season: July to October.

Medicinal uses: Has antibacterial and antiviral effects, treats diseases caused by Staphylococcus aureus (acne, impetigo, boils, cellulitis, carbuncles, staphylococcal scalded skin syndrome, abscess, pneumonia, meningitis, osteomyelitis, endocarditis, toxic shock, sepsis), treats kidney diseases. It suppresses the activity of the influenza and HIV virus. Has antioxidant, anti-inflammatory and hemostatic effects. It strengthens the reproductive organs.

Lycoperdon pyriforme - Pear-Shaped Puffball

Edible when young, when the flesh is white and elastic. It grows in large groups or rarely solitary, on decaying wood, tree trunks, wood debris (particularly after forest fires) in mixed and coniferous forests. Season: July to October.

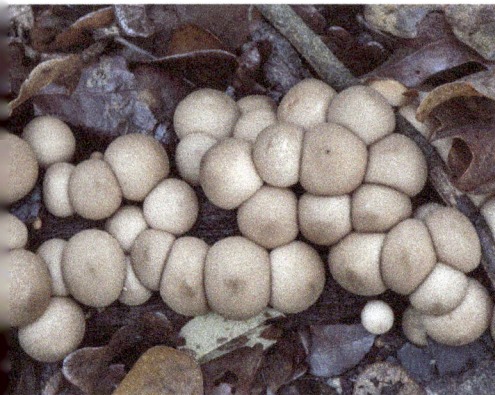

Medicinal uses: Has antibacterial, anti-inflammatory (abscesses, furunculosis), and wound-healing effects (wounds, bruises), treats diseases caused by Staphylococcus aureus (acne, impetigo, boils, cellulitis, carbuncles, staphylococcal scalded skin syndrome, abscess, pneumonia, meningitis, osteomyelitis, endocarditis, toxic shock, sepsis). Has suppressing effect on hay bacillus and has antifungal effects, used for the treatment of allergic bronchopulmonary aspergillosis. It can be used for the treatment of intestinal, paroxysmal and septic escherichiosis and frostbite.

60

Lyophyllum decastes - Clustered Domecap

Edible. The mushroom has a delicious taste. It grows in large groups and very rarely on its own in deciduous and mixed forests, along forest roadsides, in gardens, parks, meadows, and in the grass. Season: August to November.

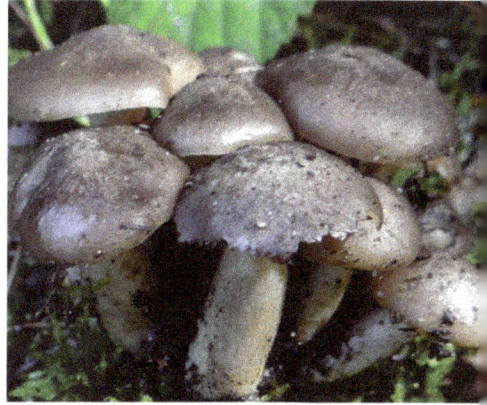

Medicinal uses: Enhances the immune system, activates anti-tumor protective systems of the body. Used to prevent and treat malignant tumors and benign formations. It provides an immuno-stimulating and immuno-modulating action. Has antihypertensive effects and hypolipidemic properties. It can be used for the prevention and treatment of diabetes mellitus and to lower cholesterol in the blood.

Lysurus mokusin - Lantern Stinkhorn

Edible when it is in the immature stage of "egg." It grows in small groups or solitary on wood waste, on shredded wood, and on compost. Season: August to November.

Medicinal uses: Has antibacterial effects, used for the treatment of non-healing wounds and ulcers. It strengthens the immune system, activates the anti-tumor protective systems of the body. Used for the prevention and treatment of malignant tumors and benign formations. It can be used to treat diseases of the gastrointestinal tract and diseases of the liver, kidneys and pancreas. It treats sexual dysfunction in men and women. Used as an aphrodisiac and to treat infertility. Has adaptogenic effect under stress. Used in gerontology, as it is thought to slow down the aging process.

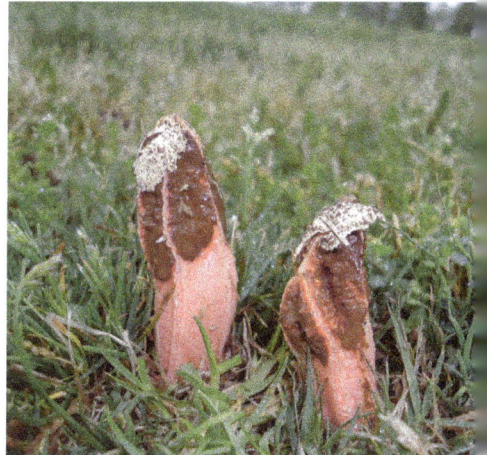

61

Macrolepiota procera - Parasol Mushroom

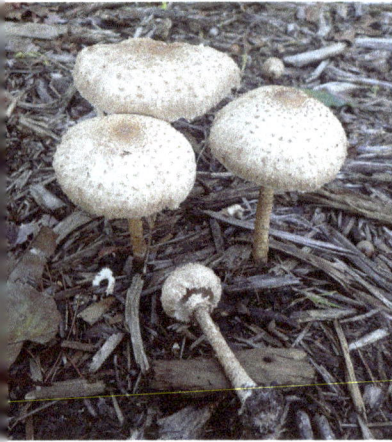

Edible. A delicacy. It grows solitary or in small groups in mixed light forests on rich soil, sometimes forming "witch circles." Can also be found on forest edges, glades, on roadsides, in fields, gardens, parks, on open grassy places, on rotted debris, on wood shavings or wood chips. Season: June to November.

Medicinal uses: Has antibacterial effects, used to treat purulent wounds. It normalizes fat metabolism and treats obesity. It improves brain activity and strengthens the nervous system. Used in cosmetology (removes puffiness, rejuvenates, tones, nourishes skin), stimulates the production of hormones. Improves functioning of the gastrointestinal tract. Used to prevent and treat gout. The mushroom normalizes cholesterol and blood circulation, improves blood composition, lowers blood sugar, strengthens and cleans blood vessels and is used to treat cardiovascular diseases.

Macrolepiota rachodes - Shaggy Parasol Mushroom

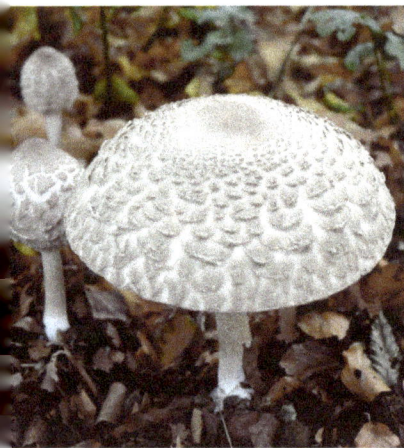

Edible. The mushroom is very tasty, reminiscent of chicken. It grows in small groups on humus soils in mixed forests, on glades, in parks, on wood shavings or wood chips, on prairie, prefers open spaces. Season: July to November.

Medicinal uses: Has antibacterial effects, used to treat purulent wounds. It improves brain activity and strengthens the nervous system. It normalizes fat metabolism and treats obesity. Has antioxidant effects, normalizes blood circulation, improves blood composition. Used to treat cardiovascular diseases. Has immuno-stimulating and immuno-modulating effects, strengthens and cleans blood vessels. Enhances the immune system, activates anti-tumor protective systems of the body.

62

Marasmius alliaceus - Garlic Parachute

Edible. The mushroom has a strong smell of garlic and is used as a seasoning. It grows in small groups or solitary on wood waste, and in moss in deciduous forests (such as birch trees). Season: July to October.

Medicinal uses: Has antibacterial and antifungal effects, enhances the immune system, activates anti-tumor protective systems of the body. Used for the prevention and treatment of malignant tumors and benign formations.

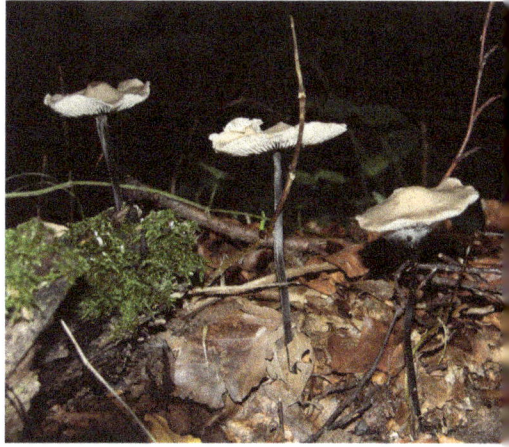

Marasmius oreades - Scotch Bonnet

Edible. Grows in small groups or solitary on lawns, gardens, on forest edges, forest glades, meadows, ravines, ditches, pastures, field margins, and roadsides, often forming arcs, rows or "fairy rings." Season: May to November or year-round in a warm climate.

Medicinal uses: Has antibacterial and antiviral effects, treats diseases caused by Staphylococcus aureus (acne, impetigo, boils, cellulitis, carbuncles, staphylococcal scalded skin syndrome, abscess, pneumonia, meningitis, osteomyelitis, endocarditis, toxic shock, sepsis), treats intestinal, paroxysmal and septic escherichiosis. Used for cosmetic purposes (skin care, acne, wrinkles, has a rejuvenating effect). Treats

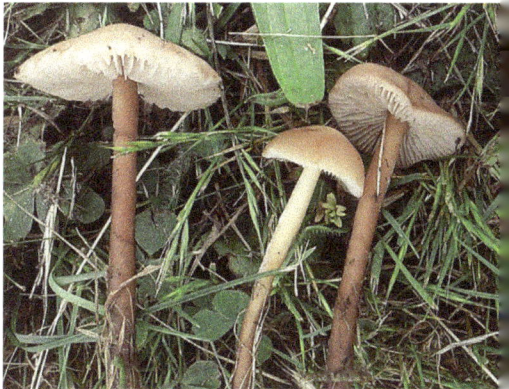

thrombosis. Can be used for the treatment of diseases affecting the endocrine and thyroid glands. Has anesthetic effects and treats muscle pains, seizures, pain in the tendons, numbness of the limbs, lumbago.

Meripilus giganteus - Giant Polypore

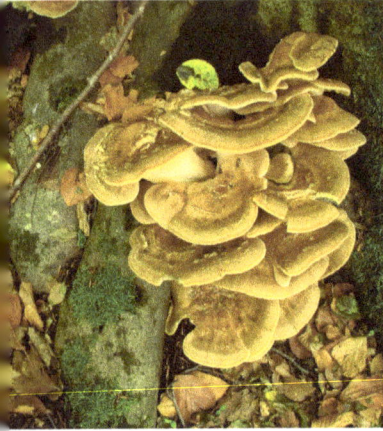

Edible when young. It grows in groups in deciduous forests, rarely in coniferous ones, on the trunks and roots of decomposing wood residue. It parasitizes on birch and sometimes on oak trees, causing a white rot. It can be found on trees in city parks. Season: August to September, or all year round in a warm climate.

Medicinal uses: Strengthens the immune system, activates anti-tumor protective systems of the body. Used for the prevention and treatment of malignant tumors and benign formations.

Morchella deliciosa - White morel

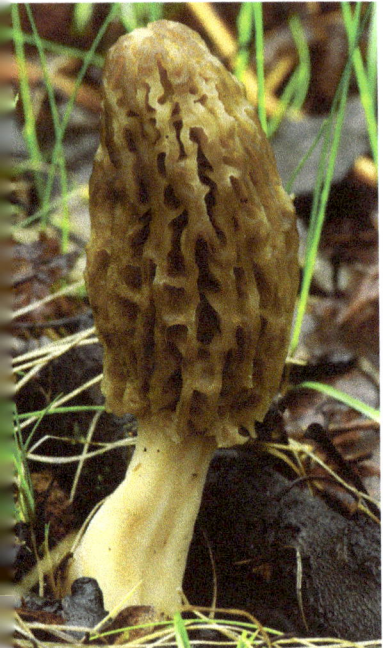

Edible when young. Highly valued by connoisseurs. It grows solitary or in groups in deciduous and coniferous forests, in gardens, under fruit trees, in parks, beside woodland tracks, forest edges, on the banks of streams, along ditches, clearings, glades, in old burned-down areas. Season: March to June, in warm areas year around.

Medicinal uses: Has antibacterial, antiviral and anti-inflammatory effects (abscesses, furunculosis), treats diseases of the respiratory system (inflammation, bronchitis, acute respiratory viral infection, influenza, etc.). Has antioxidant effects, treats eye diseases involving reduced vision (nearsightedness, farsightedness, cataracts, glaucoma). Provides immuno-stimulating and immuno-modulating action; treats joint diseases (arthrosis, arthritis, rheumatism, polyarthritis, osteochondrosis, psoriatic arthritis). It can be used for the prevention and treatment of gastrointestinal diseases. The mushroom normalizes metabolism and can be used as restorative remedy.

Morchella elata - Black Morel

Edible when young. A delicacy. It grows solitary or in groups in light deciduous forests, beside woodland tracks, forest edges, on the banks of streams, along ditches, clearings, on glades, in old burned-down areas. Season: March to June.

Medicinal uses: Has antibacterial, antiviral and anti-inflammatory effects, treats joint diseases (arthrosis, arthritis, rheumatism, polyarthritis, osteochondrosis, psoriatic arthritis) and diseases of the respiratory system. It can be used for the prevention and treatment of gastrointestinal diseases. Has antioxidant effects, normalizes metabolism and is used as restorative remedy. It provides an immuno-stimulating and immuno-modulating action, and treats eye diseases.

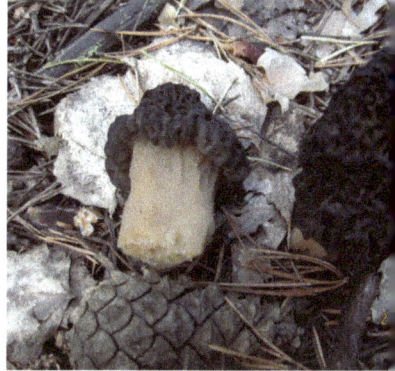

Morchella esculenta - Common Morel

Edible when young. Highly valued by connoisseurs. It grows solitary or in groups in light deciduous or mixed forests, in parks, in apple orchards, forest edges, on the banks of streams, along ditches, clearings, glades, in old burned-down areas, on lawns with fertile lime-rich soils. Season: May to September or from February to October in a warm climate.

Medicinal uses: Has antibacterial, antiviral and anti-inflammatory effects; treats diseases of the respiratory system and joint diseases. It provides an immuno-stimulating and immuno-modulating action, used for the prevention and treatment of gastrointestinal diseases. Has antioxidant effects and treats eye diseases. The mushroom normalizes metabolism and can be used as restorative remedy.

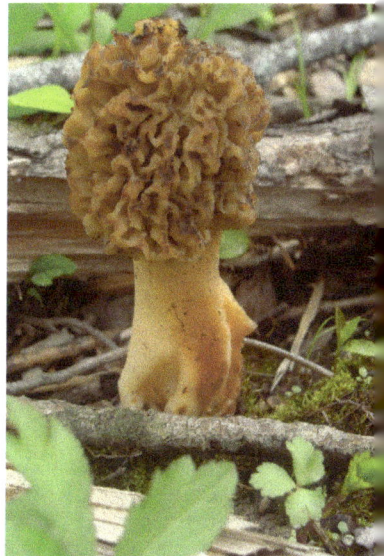

Neolentinus lepideus - Scaly Sawgill

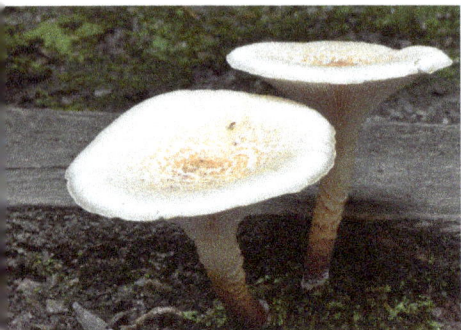

Edible. It is a parasite that grows in coniferous forests, preferring pine forests. It is also found in gardens, on flower beds, on railway sleepers, and even in closed coal mines. Rarely found in mixed forests. It decays the wood, causing wet rot. Season: April to October.

Medicinal use: Activates anti-tumor protective systems of the body, strengthens and enhances the immune system. It can be used for the prevention and treatment of malignant tumors and benign formations.

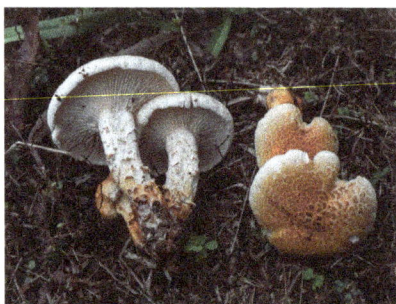

Neolentinus ponderosus - Giant Sawgill

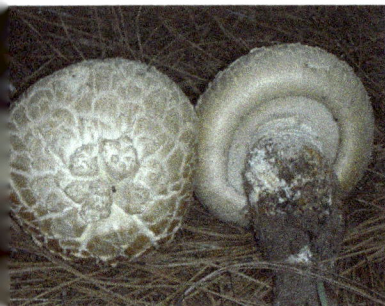

Edible when young and fresh. It grows in small groups on decaying wood, on stumps and logs, on dead trees in deciduous and coniferous forests, preferring Ponderosa pine, causes brown rot. Season: usually May to September.

Medicinal uses: Has antiviral effects, suppresses the activity of influenza and HIV viruses. Used to strengthen and enhance the immune system. Activates the anti-tumor protective systems of the body and is used for the prevention and treatment of malignant tumors and benign formations.

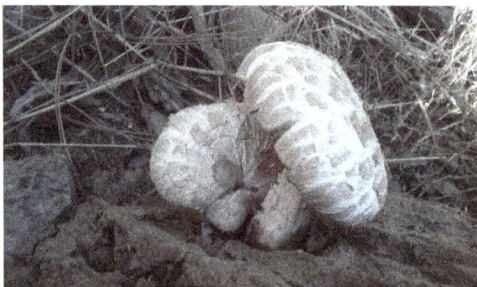

Panellus serotinus - Late Oyster

Edible. Grows in groups on decaying wood, on stumps, remains of various hardwoods, preferring deciduous trees (maple, aspen, elm, linden, birch and poplar) and less common on coniferous trees. Season: September to December.

Medicinal uses: Activates anti-tumor protective systems of the body, strengthens and enhances the immune system. Has antioxidant effects. Used for the prevention and treatment of diabetes mellitus. It provides an immuno-stimulating and immuno-modulating action. It can be used for the prevention and treatment of malignant tumors and benign formations.

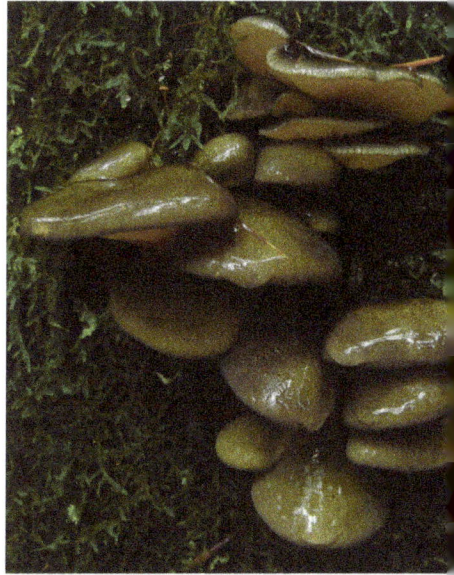

Paxillus atrotomentosus - Velvet Roll-Rim

Conditionally edible. Grows solitary or in small groups on decaying wood trunks of deciduous and coniferous trees, on stumps, logs, wood residue, and in the moss. Season: July to October.

Medicinal use: Has analgesic effects, treats muscle pain, cramps, pain in the tendons,

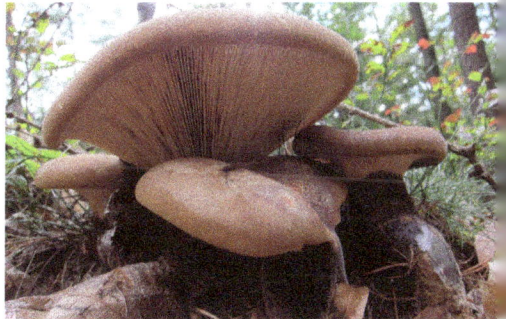

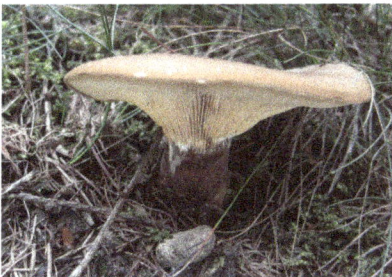

numbness of the limbs, lumbago. It strengthens and enhances the immune system and activates anti-tumor protective systems of the body. Used for the prevention and treatment of malignant tumors and benign formations.

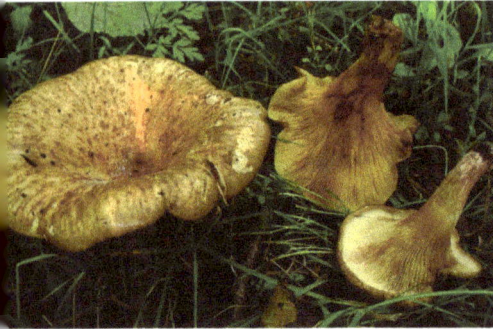

Conditionally edible. Grows solitary or in groups on the ground in deciduous and mixed forests, forming mycorrhiza with alder or aspen. It can be found across the Northern Hemisphere. Season: July to October.

Medicinal use: Strengthens and enhances the immune system. Has analgesic effects, treats muscle pain, cramps, pain in the tendons, numbness of the limbs, lumbago. It can be used for the prevention and treatment of benign formations and malignant tumors.

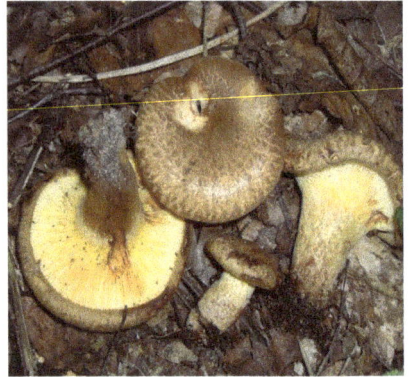

Peziza badia - Bay Cup

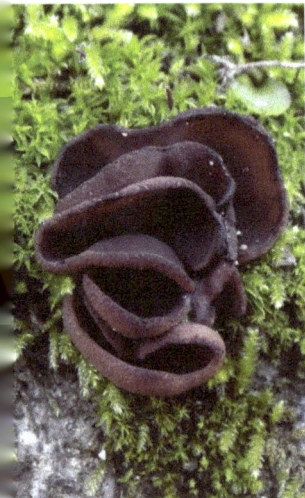

Edible. Grows on weakened or dead deciduous trees and bushes. It occurs solitary or in small groups in broad-leaf or conifer forests, on fallen trees, rotten wood and on the ground. Season: April to October, all year round in warm areas.

Medicinal uses:
Provides an immuno-stimulating and immuno-modulating action, enhances the immune system, activates anti-tumor protective systems of the body. Used to treat and prevent malignant tumors and benign formations.

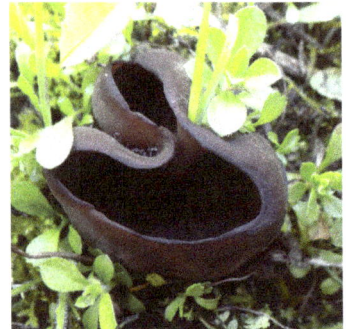

Peziza vesiculosa - Blistered Cup

Edible. Grows in small groups on fertile ground mixed with manure, on rotting sheaves of straw or on manure heaps. Season: June to September, in warm areas, all year round.

Medicinal uses: Has hemostatic and anti-inflammatory effects, treats cardiovascular diseases, thrombosis and varicose veins. It provides immuno-stimulating and immuno-modulating action and removes toxins from the body. It enhances the functioning of the gastrointestinal tract. Used for the prevention and treatment of allergies. Has pain relief effects, normalizes the body's metabolism, improves vision and treats obesity. It helps cope with seasickness.

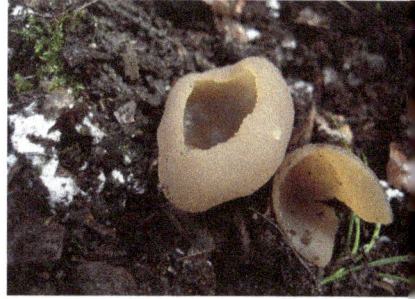

Phallus impudicus - Common Stinkhorn

Edible when the mushroom is in the immature stage of "egg." It grows solitary in deciduous and coniferous forests in humus-rich soils, as well as in parks and gardens. It forms mycorrhiza with beech and oak trees and some shrubs. The spores are spread by insects. It can be grown in any backyard. Season: May to October.

Medicinal uses: Has antibacterial, antiviral and anti-inflammatory effects, treats herpes, colds, influenza, typhoid, and para-typhoid. Provides immuno-stimulating and immuno-modulating action, treats pulmonary tuberculosis, diabetes mellitus and endocrine gland diseases. Has antioxidant and analgesic effects, treats joint diseases, post-stroke conditions, paralysis. It can be used to treat atherosclerosis, treats eye diseases and improves vision. It treats sexual dysfunction of men and women. Used as aphrodisiac and to treat infertility. Has adaptogenic effect under stress. Used in gerontology, as it is said to slow down the aging process.

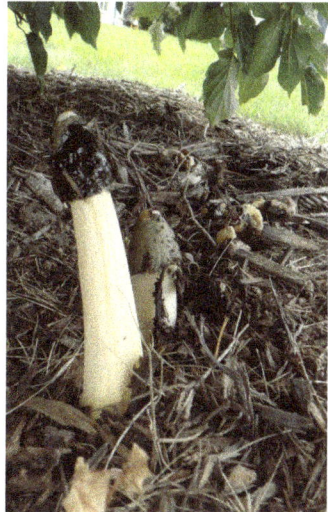

Phellinus igniarius - False Tinder

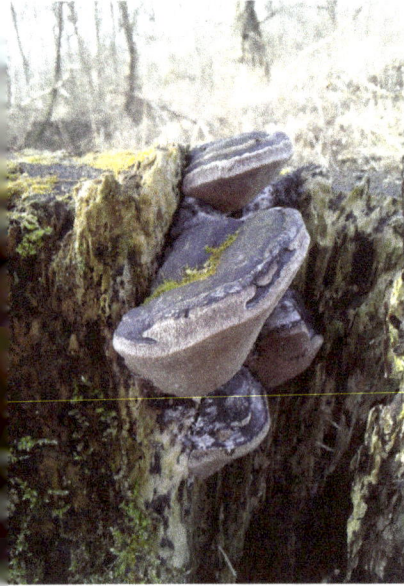

Inedible. Parasitizes and grows on the trunks of hardwood (especially willow trees), as well as on stumps, damaged or dead trees. Living trees are infected through damage to the bark, broken branches, cracks. A healing tea is prepared from the fungus. Season: all year round.

Medicinal uses: Has strong antibacterial and anti-inflammatory effects. Used for the treatment of sore throat, festering and non-healing wounds.

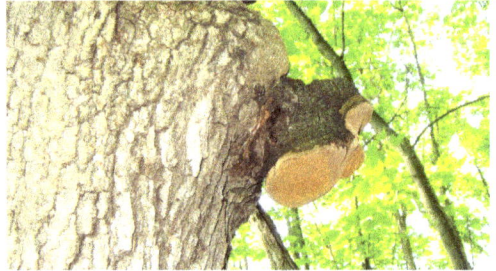

Pholiota lubrica - Scale Slippery

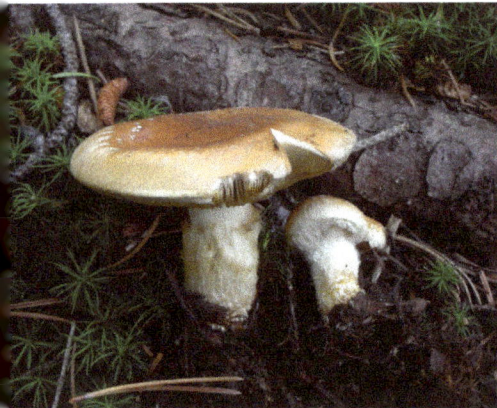

Conditionally edible. Must be boiled for 10 minutes in water, then drained, after which it can be used in dishes. Grows in small groups or colonies in mixed and deciduous forests on humus-rich soils, on wood residues (birch, oak), and around stumps. Season: August to October.

Medicinal uses: Has antibacterial effect, treats non-healing wounds. Used to lower cholesterol level.

70

Piptoporus betulinus - Birch Polypore

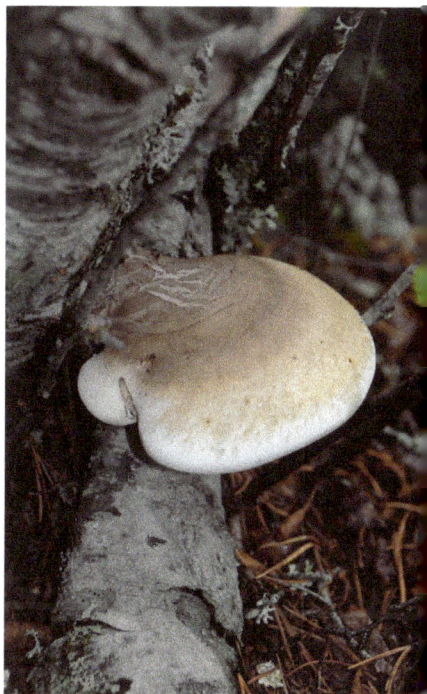

Inedible. It grows parasitically in groups or solitary on the trunks of weakened or dead birch trees. A tree infected by the fungi breaks down very quickly, becoming rotten from within. The mushroom caps develop on the rotten wood of the trunk. A healing tea is prepared from the fungus. Season: all year round.

Medicinal uses: Has antibacterial, antiviral and anti-inflammatory effects (abscesses, boils), treats intestinal, par- oxysmal and septic escherichiosis. Used as an antihilmintic agent (entero-biosis, teniosis, trichocephalus, asca-riasis, nematodes, giardiasis, schistoso-miasis, opisthorchiasis, clonorchiasis). Provides an immuno-stimulating and immuno-modulating action. Used for the treatment of tick-borne encephalitis. It normalizes metabolism and is used as a restorative remedy.

Pleurotus dryinus - Veiled Oyster

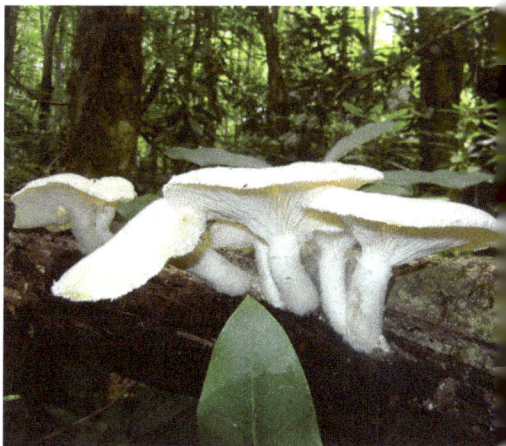

Edible. Grows and parasitizes on the trunks of weakened or dead. Grows in small groups or soli-tary on trunks of dead oaks and other deciduous trees. In some countries it is included in the Red Book. Season: July to October.

Medicinal uses: Strengthens the immune system, activates the anti-tumor protective systems of the body. Used for the prevention and treatment of malignant tu-mors and benign formations.

71

Pleurotus giganteus - Swine's Stomach

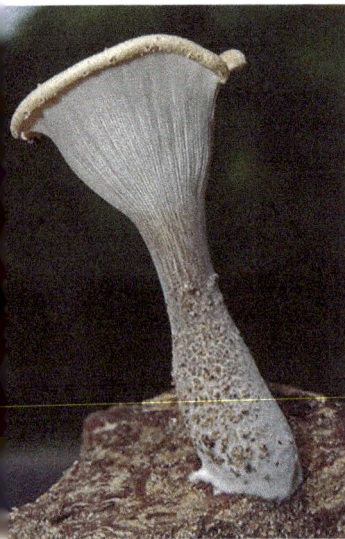

Edible when young and fresh. It grows in large groups on decaying wood, on stumps, dried or weakened trunks of deciduous trees (birch, oak, mountain ash, willow, aspen), sometimes found on coniferous species or on fallen and dry trees and can even be found in parks or gardens. Season: May to December or all year round in warm climate.

Medicinal uses: Has antimutagenic and antioxidant effects, treats diseases of the nervous system. Has hepatoprotective activities, treats candidiasis (thrush). Can be used for the mitigation of neurodegenerative diseases, treats Alzheimer's disease, Parkinson's disease, Huntington's disease, senile dementia.

Pleurotus ostreatus - Oyster Mushroom

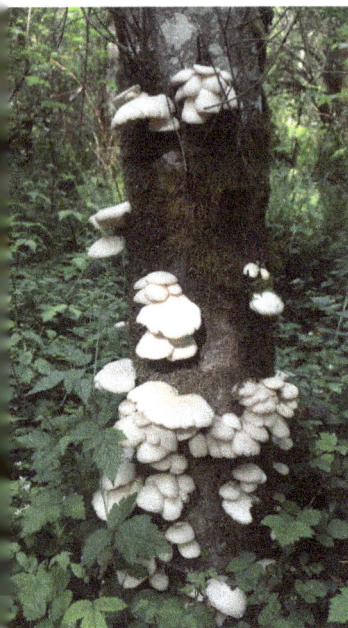

Edible when young and fresh. It surpasses vegetables and meat for its valuable qualities. It grows in large groups on decaying wood, on stumps, dried or weakened trunks of deciduous trees (birch, oak, rowan, willow, aspen), on fallen trees, dead wood, in parks and gardens, sometimes found on conifers. Season: May to December or all year round in warm climate.

Medicinal uses: Has antiviral and antitoxic effects, used for the treatment of HIV infection. The mushroom is used to treat diseases of the nervous system. Has analgesic effects, treats muscle pain, cramps, pain in the tendons, numbness of the limbs, lumbago. Has anti-mutagenic and antioxidant effects. It can be used for the treatment of cardiovascular diseases and hypertension, to lower cholesterol level.

Pleurotus populinus - Aspen Oyster

Edible when young and fresh. It grows mostly in large groups on decaying wood, on stumps, dried trunks of deciduous trees (aspen, black cottonwood), on fallen trees, dead wood, and can sometimes be found in aspen groves in city parks and gardens. Season: May to July.

Medicinal uses: Has antiviral and antitoxic effects, used for the treatment of HIV infection. It can be used to treat diseases of the nervous system. Has analgesic effects, treats muscle pain, cramps, pain in the tendons, numbness of the limbs, lumbago. Has antimutagenic and antioxidant effects, treats cardiovascular diseases and hypertension, and lowers cholesterol level.

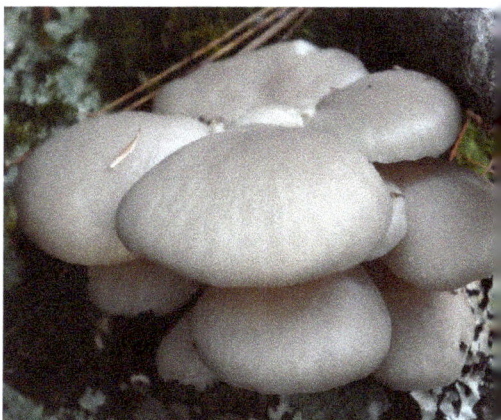

Pleurotus pulmonarius - Lung Oyster

Edible. Grows in large groups or solitary on decaying wood, weakened trees and stumps, hardwood trunks (birch, aspen, poplar, willow, beech, alder, linden, etc.), causing white rot. Season: May to October. In warm climates, it grows all year round.

Medicinal uses: Has antibacterial effects. Used for prevention and treatment of diabetes mellitus. Has anesthetic and antioxidant effects, used to treat hay fever, lowers cholesterol level.

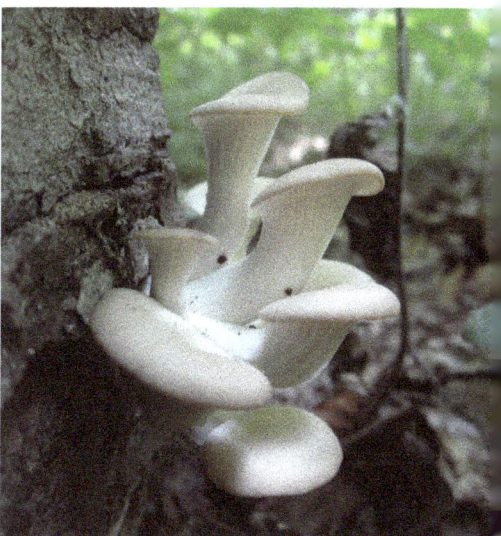

Pluteus cervinus - Deer Shield

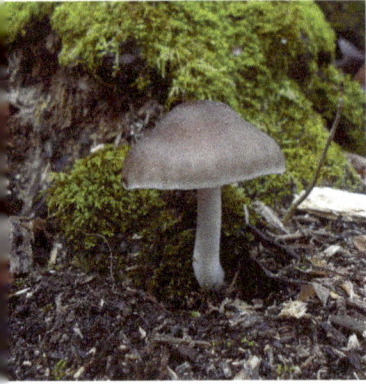

Edible. Grows solitary or in small groups on decaying wood, around stumps, on fallen trees, on the remains of bark, on sawdust, wood chips, and in forest clearings in deciduous, and rarely, coniferous forests. Season: May to October.

Medicinal uses: Enhances the immune system, activates the anti-tumor protective systems of the body. Used for the prevention and treatment of malignant tumors and benign formations, treats thrombosis.

Polyozellus multiplex - Black Chanterelle

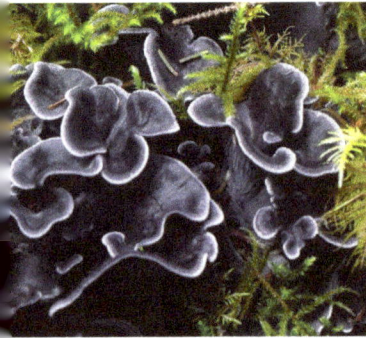

Edible. Grows in small groups or solitary in coniferous forests, mainly under pine and spruce trees. Season: spring to fall.

Medicinal uses: Enhances the immune system, activates the anti-tumor protective systems of the body. Used for the prevention and treatment of malignant tumors (stomach cancer) and benign formations. The mushroom can be used for the prevention and treatment of Alzheimer's disease and senile dementia.

Polyporus alveolaris - Hexagonal-pored Polypore

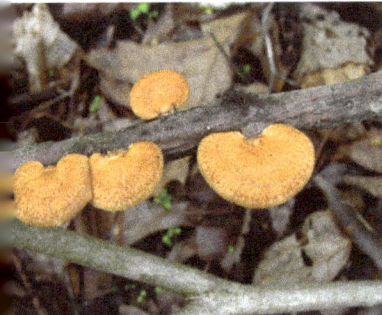

Edible when young. Grows solitary or in small groups on decaying wood debris of deciduous trees. Season: April to August.

Medicinal uses: Strengthens the immune system, activates the anti-tumor protective systems of the body. Used for prevention and treatment of malignant tumors and benign formations.

Polyporus squamosus - Dryad's Saddle

Edible when young. It grows parasitically, solitarily or in small groups on the trunks of elms, birches, sycamores and other deciduous trees, causing white rot. Season: May to September.

Medicinal uses: Enhances the immune system. Used for prevention and treatment of malignant tumors and benign formations, activates the anti-tumor protective systems of the body.

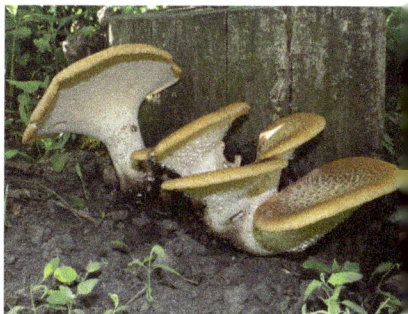

Poria cocos - Indian Bread

Edible. The mushroom has a tubular shape. Grows underground on the wet roots of the high-mountain pines (Pinus massoniana, Pinus densiflora, Pinus thunbergii, Pinus yunnanensis, Pinus taiwanensis, Pinus longifolis, etc.) and on their rotten stumps. Season: June to October.

Medicinal uses: Has antibacterial and anti-inflammatory effects, treats catarrhs, bronchitis, and tracheitis, relieves cough and helps with sputum removal, treats lungs and bronchial tubes. It prevents the development of metastasis, reduces the toxic effects of chemotherapy, removes toxins from the body, prevents the destruction of red blood cells by cancer. Used as a restorative remedy. It helps with swelling and the prevention and treatment of edema of renal and cardiac origin. It can be used for stimulation and strengthening of the circulatory system and the heart muscle. Improves the metabolism and water balance in the body. It helps the body recover after strenuous physical activity and mental exhaustion. Used as tonic and sedative after a stroke. It heals nervousness, neurasthenia, insomnia. It can be used for the activation of central nervous system functions in encephalopathies of various origins. Treats depression. It restores and improves intestinal digestion (bloating, diarrhea, indigestion). Treats diseases of the bladder. Helps dissolve kidney stones and has a protective effect on the kidneys. Stimulates the stomach, spleen, liver. It strengthens the body during aging too, and has adaptogenic effects when under stress.

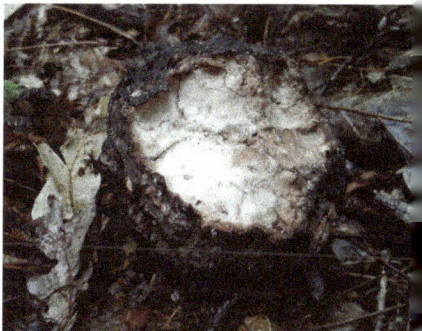

Psathyrella candolleana - Pale Brittlestem

Conditionally edible. Must be boiled for 10 minutes in water, then drained, after which it can be used in dishes. Grows in groups in meadows and pastures, on the debris of deciduous trees, around stumps, sometimes on live trees. Season: May to October.

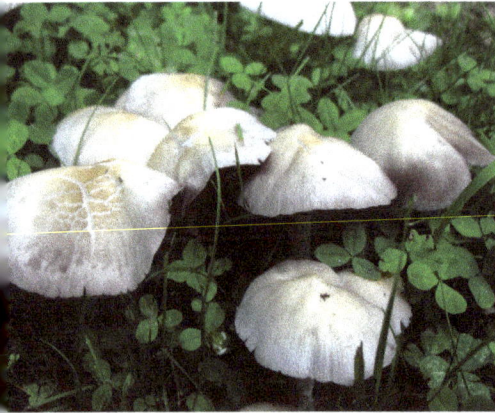

Medicinal uses: Has antibacterial effects, treats diseases caused by Staphylococcus aureus (acne, impetigo, boils, cellulitis, carbuncles, staphylococcal scalded skin syndrome, abscess, pneumonia, meningitis, osteomyelitis, endocarditis, toxic shock, sepsis). Has a suppressing effect on hay bacillus. It treats food poisoning (including vomiting and diarrhea symptoms), salmonellosis. Has antifungal effect, used for the treatment of candidiasis (thrush).

Pseudohydnum gelatinosum - Toothed Jelly Fungus

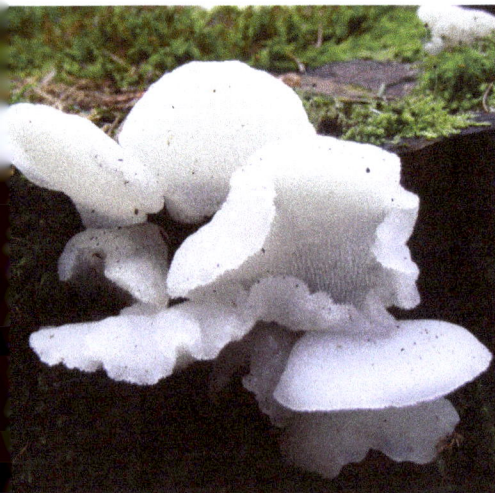

Edible. Grows in groups or solitary in forests of various types, prefers the remains of deciduous, but more often coniferous trees on wood residues, on wet stumps, on trunks of pine trees and even eucalyptus trees. It is rare. Season: September to October.

Medicinal uses: Enhances the immune system, activates the anti-tumor protective systems of the body. Used for the prevention and treatment of malignant tumors and benign formations.

Pycnoporus sanguineus - Cinnabar Bracket

Inedible. Grows in groups or solitary on wood residue, wet stumps, trunks of various trees and on decaying branches, roots, and fallen trees. Season: all year round.

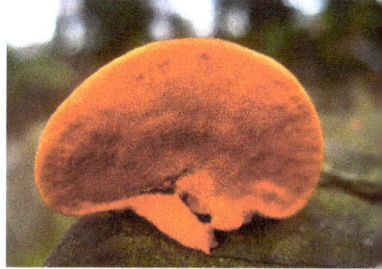

Medicinal uses: Has antibacterial effects. Used for the treatment of sore throat and non-healing wounds and ulcers. The mushroom facilitates the removal of heavy metals from the body. Has an anti-hemorrhagic effect on hemorrhages. It can be used to treat fever and toothache, treats arthritis and gout.

Ramaria botrytis - Clustered Coral

Edible when young and fresh. Grows solitary or in large groups in mixed and deciduous forests, mainly near beeches, less often under coniferous species of trees. Season: June to October.

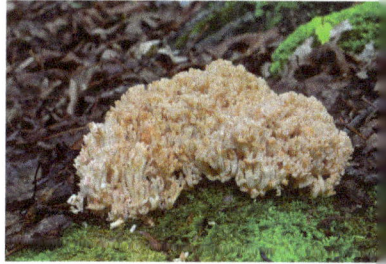

Medicinal uses: Has antibacterial and anti-inflammatory effects (abscesses, furunculosis), treats sore throat, rheumatism, acute glomerulonephritis, streptococcal toxic shock syndrome and postpartum sepsis. Has analgesic effects and can be used for the treatment of muscle pain, seizures, pain in the tendons, numbness of the limbs, lumbago. It treats liver diseases and listeriosis.

Russula aurea - Gilded Brittlegill

Edible. Found in small groups on forest edges, clearings, among the moss, and on roadsides. It grows in coniferous and deciduous forests. Season: June to October.

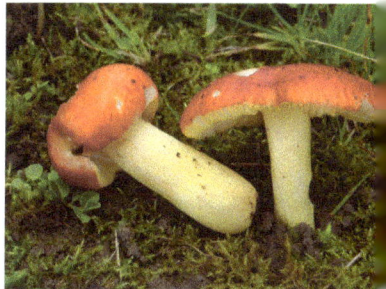

Medicinal uses: Helps cleanse the stomach and intestines. Used for the prevention and treatment of atherosclerosis and obesity.

Russula cyanoxantha - Charcoal Burner

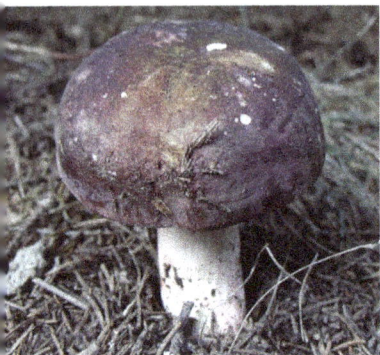

Edible. This mushroom is highly regarded among gourmets. It grows in mixed and deciduous forests (especially birch), on the edges, clearings, among the moss, and on roadsides. Season: May to November, with the best growth from July to September.

Medicinal uses: Used for prevention and treatment of atherosclerosis and obesity. Has an antioxidant effect and helps cleanse the stomach and intestines.

Russula delica - Milk-white Brittlegill

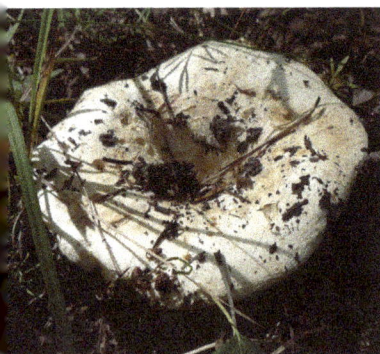

Edible. Grows in edges and clearings of coniferous, mixed and deciduous forests (especially under birch, aspen, fir, oak, beech, pine, alder). It forms mycorrhiza with deciduous trees, mainly with birch and aspen. Season: June to November.

Medicinal uses: Enhances the immune system, activates the anti-tumor protective systems of the body. Used for the prevention and treatment of malignant tumors and benign formations.

Russula fragilis - Fragile Brittlegill

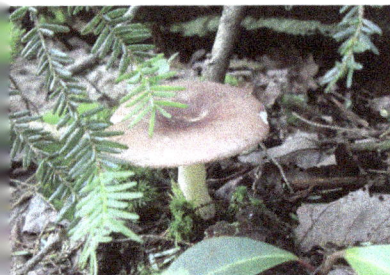

Edible. Grows in small groups or solitary in mixed and deciduous forests. Season: June to October.

Medicinal uses: Has antioxidant effects, helps cleanse the stomach and intestines. Can be used for prevention and treatment of atherosclerosis and to lower cholesterol, treats obesity.

Russula graveolens - Russula Purpurea

Edible. Widespread on the forest edges and clearings of coniferous, mixed and deciduous forests. Season: June to October.

Medicinal uses: Helps cleanse the stomach and intestines. Used for the prevention and treatment of atherosclerosis, obesity.

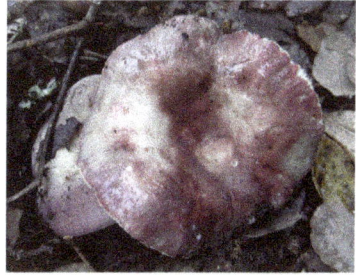

Russula lepida - Rosy Russula

Edible. Grows in mixed and deciduous forests (especially birch), on the edges, among the moss, and on roadsides. Season: May to November, greatest growth from July to October.

Medicinal uses: Has antioxidant effects, used for prevention and treatment of atherosclerosis and obesity. It helps cleanse the stomach and intestines.

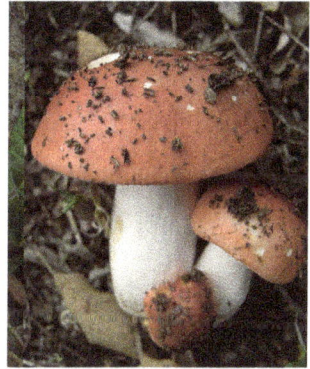

Russula virescens - Green-cracking Russula

Edible. Considered to be one of the best in the Russulaceae family. Grows in mixed and deciduous forests mainly under oak, beech, birch, aspen trees. Season: June to October.

Medicinal uses: Has antioxidant and antibacterial effects. Used for the prevention and treatment of atherosclerosis, obesity, and to lower cholesterol. Helps cleanse the stomach and intestines.

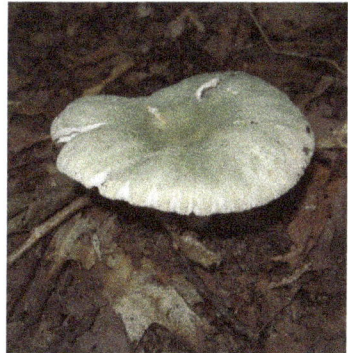

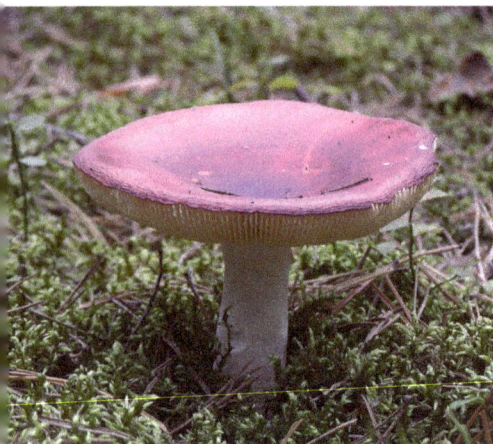

Edible. Considered a delicacy. It grows solitary or in groups in coniferous and mixed forests, mainly under oak, birch, fir, pine or larch trees. Season: June to October.

Medicinal uses: Helps cleanse the stomach and intestines. Used for prevention and treatment of atherosclerosis. It normalizes fat metabolism and treats obesity. The fungus has anti-parasitic activity and treats malaria.

Sarcodon imbricatus - Shingled Hedgehog

Edible when young. It grows in large groups or solitary, on sandy dry soils in coniferous forests, forming mycorrhiza with pine, less often with other coniferous trees and sometimes forming "witch circles." The mushroom has an unusual spicy smell. The mushroom rarely can be found in mixed forests. Season: August to November.

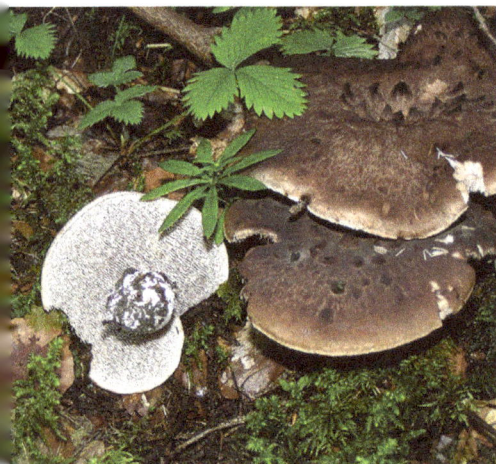

Medicinal uses: Has antibacterial effects. Used for the treatment of diseases caused by Staphy- lococcus aureus (acne, impetigo, boils, cellulitis, carbuncles, staphylococcal scalded skin syndrome, abscess, pneumonia, meningitis, osteomyelitis, endocarditis, sepsis, infectious-toxic shock). It treats hospital-acquired infections. Has a suppressing effect on hay bacillus. It provides an immuno-stimulating and immuno- modulating action. Lowers cholesterol level.

Edible when young. It is considered to be a delicacy in tropical countries. It grows solitary or in small groups on decaying wood residue of coniferous and deciduous trees. Season: spring to autumn.

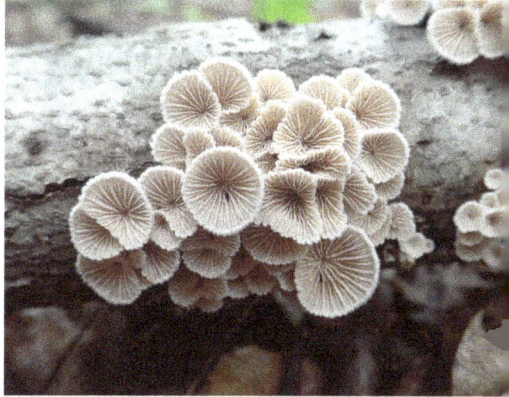

Medicinal uses: Has antibacterial, antiviral and anti-inflammatory effects. Treats diseases caused by Staphylococcus aureus and diseases caused by HIV. It can be used for prevention and treatment of infectious diseases of the reproductive system, enteritis, cystitis and septic wounds. Has anti-fungal effects, treats intestinal, paroxysmal and septic escherichiosis. It provides an immuno-stimulating and immuno-modulating action, treats diseases of the lymphatic system. It normalizes metabolism and can be used as a restorative remedy. Treats chronic fatigue syndrome. Has a tonic effect on general weakness of the body and reduced tone.

Edible when young. It grows parasitically, solitary or in small groups, in coniferous and mixed forests, on the roots, often at the bases of trunks, sometimes on freshly cut stumps. The fungus causes destructive rot of the roots and bases of trees. Season: July to October.

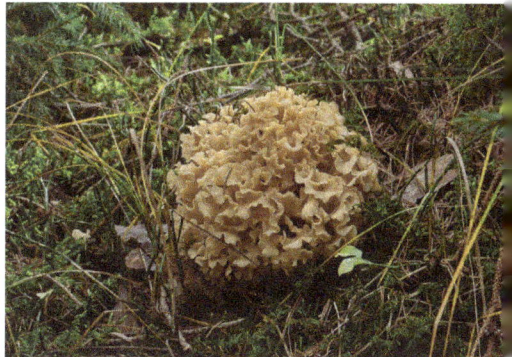

Medicinal uses: Has antibacterial and antiviral effects. Used to treat cardiovascular diseases and hypertension, and enhances hematopoiesis. Has an antifungal effect, treats intestinal, paroxysmal and septic escherichiosis. Has a suppressing effect on hay bacillus. Used for the prevention and treatment of diabetes mellitus.

Stropharia aeruginosa - Verdigris Agaric

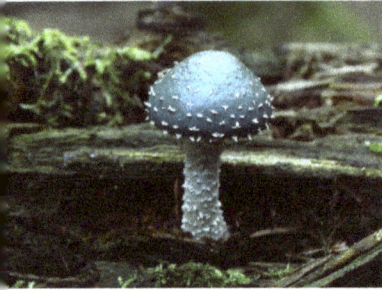

Edible. Grows solitary or in small groups in the grass, along roadsides, on decaying wood, on wood chips, as well as in the gardens, parks and pastures. Season: May to November.

Medicinal uses: Enhances the immune system, activates the anti-tumor protective systems of the body, and treats diseases of the nervous system.

Suillus granulatus - Weeping Bolete

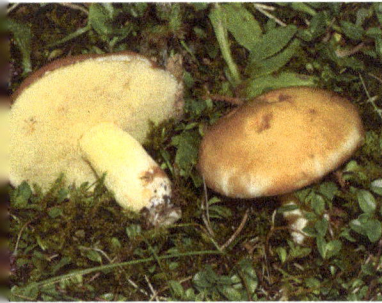

Edible. Grows in large groups or solitary in coniferous forests, forming mycorrhiza with pine. It also appears in young forests or plantations, glades, and roadsides. Season: June to November.

Medicinal uses: Has antibacterial effects, treats angina pectoris and hypertension, reduces the viscosity of blood. It helps treat headaches. Used for the prevention and treatment of gout.

Suillus luteus - Slippery Jack

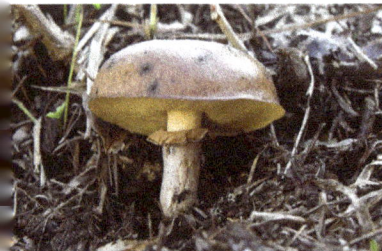

Edible. This delicious mushroom grows solitary or in large groups in pine forests and plantations, forming mycorrhiza with pine trees. It also occurs in young pine-birch or pine-oak forests and plantations, in meadows, forest edges, clearings, and roadsides, sometimes in meadows under separate trees. Season: June to October.

Medicinal uses: Has antibacterial and antiviral effects, treats diseases caused by influenza viruses, and treats Kashin-Beck disease. Used for the treatment of gout and gouty arthritis. It treats headaches (chronic arachnoiditis), migraines and heart pain. It can be used for the prevention and treatment of angina pectoris, hypertension.

Suillus placidus - Slippery White Bolete

Edible. Grows solitary or in small groups in mixed forests, together with European, Siberian and Korean cedar trees. Season: June to November.

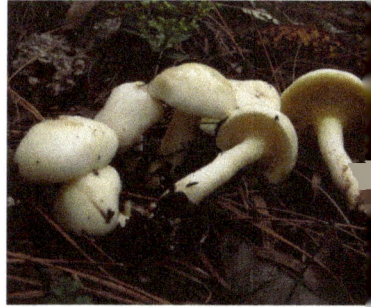

Medicinal uses: Treats gout and gouty arthritis. It can be used for the prevention and treatment of angina pectoris and hypertension. It treats headaches (chronic arachnoiditis), migraines and heart pain.

Tibetan Milk Mushroom

Inedible. This is very valuable microorganism formed during the interaction of fermented bacteria and yeast fungi (acetic acid bacteria, lactobacilli, milk yeast, etc). It has a spherical shape. In external characteristics it is similar to cottage cheese, and at a more mature age - on inflorescences of cauliflower. It is used for making sour-milk drinks. It can be grown in all countries of the world all year round.

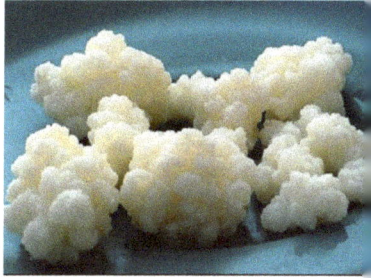

Medicinal uses: Has antibacterial, antiviral, antioxidant and anti-inflammatory effects. It removes toxins and heavy metals from the body. It helps regulate blood pressure and cholesterol level. It regulates fat metabolism and treats obesity. It slows down the aging process of the body with regular use, improves skin condition and prevents wrinkles, whitens and rejuvenates the skin, strengthens hair shafts, prevents hair loss and improves hair growth, eliminates dandruff. Tibetan Milk Mushroom helps to remove small stones from the gallbladder and kidneys. It is used to prevent infertility, restore reproductive function, improve libido and prevent the development of prostatitis. It treats cardiovascular diseases, rickets, anemia, edema, allergies. It helps with swelling of the extremities and relieves heaviness in the legs. It restores and stabilizes the natural microflora in the stomach, regulates the level of glucose in the blood and prevents the consequences of diabetes. Has a calming effect on the nervous system, relieves nerve strain, has antidepressant effects, reduces anxiety and irritability and improves mood. It enhances memory and concentration and has a tonic effect.

83

Inedible. Grows in groups or solitary on the trunks and stumps of dead hardwood (birch, oak, etc.), sometimes can be found on conifers, causes a white rot. Fruit bodies usually form large clusters which grow on top of each other or in form of rosettes. A healing tea is prepared from the fungus. Season: spring to autumn in a moderate climate. It grows all year round in warm areas.

Medicinal uses: Has strong antibacterial and antiviral effects, treats respiratory diseases (inflammation, bronchitis, SARS, influenza, acute

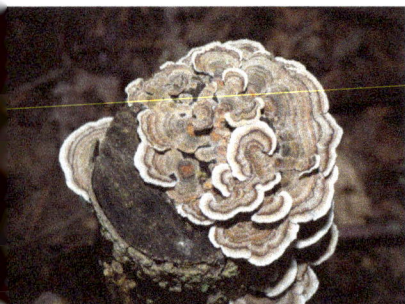

and chronic bronchitis, etc.) and diseases caused by HIV. It reduces metastasis of malignant tumors and prolongs the life of cancer patients. It can be used for the treatment of autoimmune diseases — systemic lupus erythematosus, dermatomyositis, chronic rheumatoid arthritis, multiple sclerosis. It treats gastrointestinal diseases, liver diseases (cirrhosis of the liver), and regulates and improves liver and kidney function. It provides an immuno-stimulating and immuno-modulating action. Used for the treatment of hypertension and arrhythmia, for normalization of blood pressure, for the regulation of cholesterol in the blood. It treats diseases of the lungs, intestines, kidneys and bladder, treats glomerulonephritis, diabetes mellitus, rheumatism, thrombosis. Has antifungal effects, treats candidiasis (thrush), multicolored lichen, trichophytosis (ringworm).

Tremella foliacea - Leafy Brain

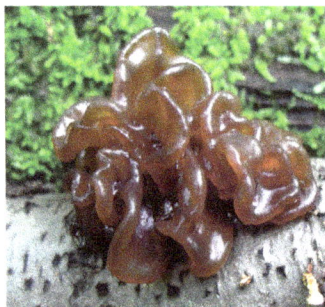

Edible. Grows in groups or solitary, on tree trunks, stumps, wood residues, and on dead fallen deciduous and coniferous trees. Season: autumn to winter.

Medicinal uses: Enhances the immune system, activates anti-tumor protective systems of the body. Used for the prevention and treatment of malignant tumors and benign formations.

Tremella fuciformis - Silver Ear Fungus

Edible. Grows in mixed forests and parasitizes together with fungi of the genus Hypoxylon and Annulohypoxylon. It can be found on trunks, stumps, wood residues, in damp places, and on fallen dead trees. Season: September to October.

Medicinal uses: Has antibacterial and anti-inflammatory effects, treats respiratory diseases (inflammation, bronchitis, SARS, influenza, etc.) and tuberculosis. It provides an immuno-stimulating and immuno-modulating action, used for the prevention and treatment of diabetes mellitus. The mushroom is used in gerontology, as it is said to slow down the aging process, and used as a cosmetic to improve the condition of the skin and smooth wrinkles. It treats gastrointestinal diseases, kidney diseases, obesity and cellulite. It can be used for the treatment of cardiovascular diseases and for normalization of blood pressure. It normalizes the body's metabolism and has a restorative effect, treats allergies. Has adaptogenic effect under stress.

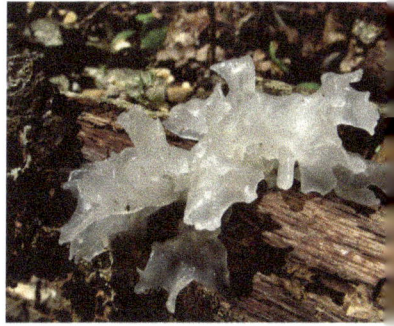

Tremella mesenterica - Golden Jelly Fungus

Edible. Grows in mixed forests and parasitizes along with mushrooms of the genus Peniophora. The mushroom can be found on trunks, stumps, wood residues, in wet places, on fallen dead trees (maple, poplar, pine, alder, etc.). Season: all year round.

Medicinal uses: Has antibacterial and anti-inflammatory effects (abscesses, furunculosis), treats respiratory diseases (inflammation, bronchitis, SARS, influenza, etc.). It provides an immuno-stimulating and immuno-modulating action. It can be used for the prevention and treatment of bronchial asthma and allergies. It treats diabetes mellitus, liver diseases and hypertension. It normalizes the body's metabolism and can be used as restorative and sedative remedy.

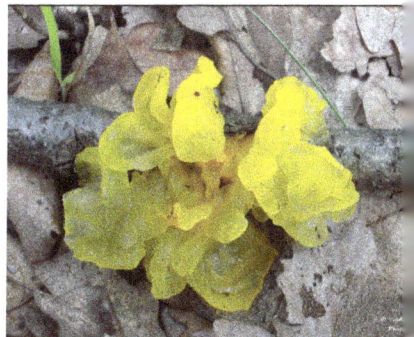

Tricholoma matsutake - Pine Mushroom

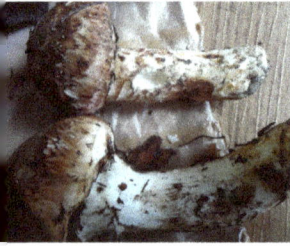

Edible. Considered a delicacy and much appreciated in Chinese, Japanese and Korean cuisine. It grows in groups, preferring dry, infertile soil in mixed and coniferous forests, forming mycorrhiza with red pine, fir, and other trees. Season: June to August.

Medicinal uses: Has antiviral effects, used for prevention and treatment of diabetes mellitus. Has sedative and analgesic effects, treats insomnia, hypertension. Has a bleaching effect on skin (treats skin dark spots).

Tricholoma portentosum - Charbonnier

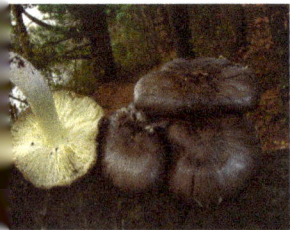

Edible. Grows solitary or in groups on sandy soils, in the moss or under wood residue in mixed and coniferous forests. The fungus forms mycorrhiza with pine, oak, birch and other trees. Season: September to October.

Medicinal uses: Has antibacterial, antifungal and antioxidant effects, treats food poisoning (including vomiting and diarrhea symptoms), and cryptococcosis. Has a suppressing effect on hay bacillus.

Tuber gibbosum – Oregon spring white truffle

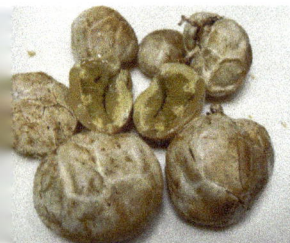

Edible. Native to the Pacific Northwest of North America. Forms mycorrhiza with coniferous trees: Douglas fir, spruce, pine, hemlock and pseudo-hemlock. Season: March to May, in good years from February to June.

Medicinal uses: Strengthens the immune system, a good aphrodisiac, returns "sexual power." Prevents inflammation of all types, helps seniors suffering from "senile infirmity", improves the condition of patients with Alzheimer's disease, regulates the hormonal system, improves eyesight and treats eye diseases, has an antioxidant effect. Used in cosmetology (rejuvenates the skin and smoothes wrinkles), treats gout, improves mood.

86

Tuber oregonense - Oregon white truffle

Edible. Native to the Pacific Northwest. This mushroom grows underground in a symbiotic relationship with Douglas fir roots. It can be found in mixed conifer forests as well, and can sometimes be found in drier forests dominated by oak and other hardwoods. Season: mid-October through March.

Medicinal uses: Strengthens the immune system. A good aphrodisiac, returns "sexual power." Prevents inflammation of all types, arthritis of all types. Used in cosmetology (rejuvenates the skin and smoothes wrinkles), treats gout, improves mood. Has a calming effect, treats nervous disorders, helps seniors suffering from "senile infirmity," improves the condition of patients with Alzheimer's disease, regulates the human hormonal system, improves eyesight, has an antioxidant effect, improves the tone of blood vessels and muscle fibers.

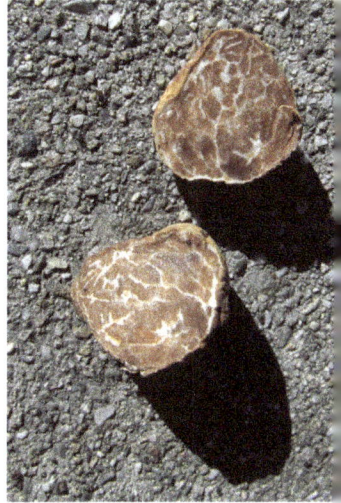

Ustilago maydis - Corn Smut

Edible. Parasitizes and grows on corn and similar species, it germinates on the flower parts, on the cob, leaves, and forms galls. Season: August to October.

Medicinal uses: Has hemostatic effect, helps to stop uterine and intestinal bleeding. Treats diseases of the female reproductive system. It improves hair growth and is used as a cosmetic agent (skincare, acne, wrinkles, rejuvenating agent). It can be used for the treatment of brain diseases (multiple sclerosis, chorea, epilepsy, vasospasm, dizziness), and psoriasis. It has antifungal effects, treats candidiasis (thrush). Used for the treatment of eye diseases with reduced vision. The mushroom has a laxative effect. It can be used for the prevention and treatment of gastrointestinal and liver diseases and as tonic remedy.

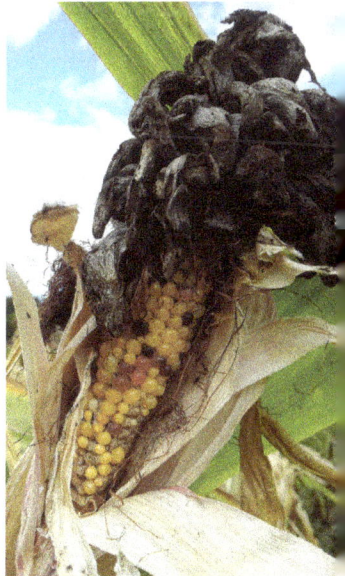

Volvariella bombycina - Silky Sheath

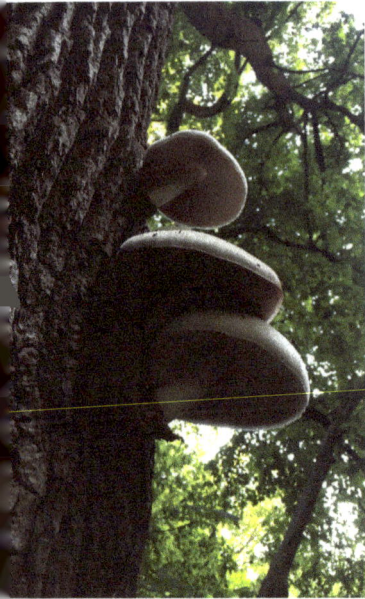

Edible. Grows solitary or in small groups on trunks and stumps of decaying deciduous trees, as well as living trees, including sugar maple, red and silver maple, magnolia, mango, birch, oak and beech trees. Sometimes this mushroom is found in coniferous forests. Season: June to October.

Medicinal uses: Has antioxidant effects, enhances the immune system, activates the anti-tumor protective systems of the body. Used for prevention and treatment of malignant tumors and benign formations. It is used as a restorative remedy after chemotherapy. The mushroom improves digestion, normalizes metabolism and promotes the removal of toxins from the body. It regulates fat metabolism and treats obesity.

Volvariella gloiocephala - Big Sheath Mushroom

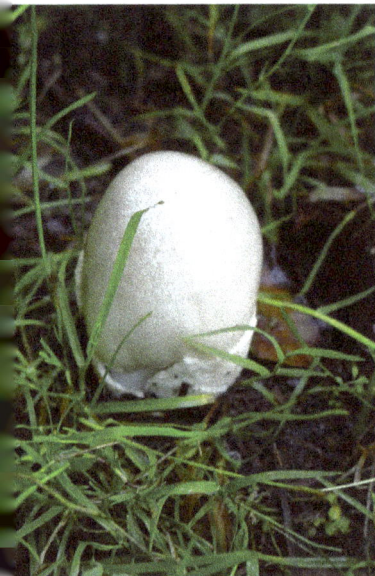

Edible. Grows in gardens, meadows, on compost and manure heaps, in greenhouses, on flower beds, on wood shavings, wood chips, or at the base of hay stacks. It is rare to find it growing in forests. Season: July to September.

Medicinal uses: Enhances the immune system, activates the anti-tumor protective systems of the body. Used for prevention and treatment of malignant tumors and benign formations. It has antibacterial, antiviral and anti-inflammatory effects. The mushroom strengthens the spleen, has a tonic effect, facilitates tolerance to summer heat. It reduces cholesterol and prevents the development of atherosclerosis. It regulates blood pressure. It can be used for the prevention and treatment of rickets and scurvy.

Volvariella volvacea - Paddy Straw Mushroom

Edible. Grows in gardens, meadows, on compost and manure heaps, in greenhouses, on flower beds, on wood chips, and near barns. Season: June to September, or in a warmer climate all year round.

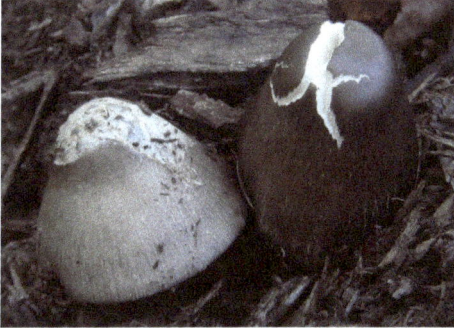

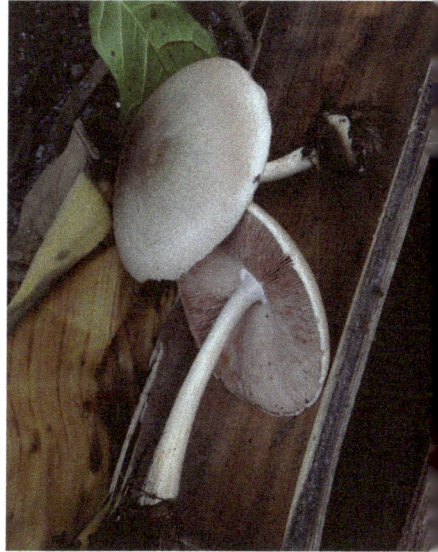

Medicinal uses: Enhances the immune system, activates anti-tumor protective systems of the body. Used for the prevention and treatment of malignant tumors and benign formations. It has antioxidant effects and can be used for the prevention and treatment of scurvy.

Xerula radicata - Deep Root Mushroom

Edible. Grows solitary or in small groups in deciduous forests, gardens, and parks on decaying wood, and on roots and trunks. It can also be found in plains and in mountains. Season: July to October.

Medicinal uses: Has antifungal effect (otomycosis), treats allergic bronchopulmonary aspergillosis, candidiasis (thrush). Used to treat of hypertension. It strengthens the immune system, activates the anti-tumor protective systems of the body. Used for prevention and treatment of malignant tumors and benign formations.

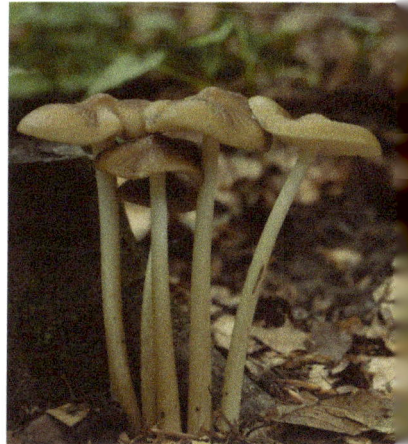

INDEX

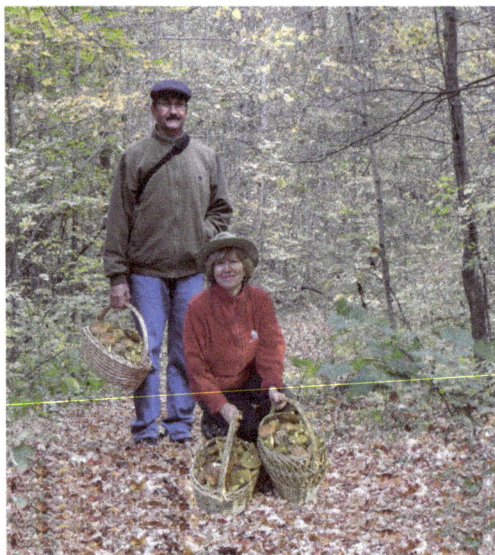

In their student years, Svetlana and Eugene Poltavets were keen on hiking, cycling and waterborne trips. Nature has always attracted them. Their fascination with medicinal plants and mushroom picking began as an amateur pursuit, but over time, they came to understand the importance of using natural remedies contained in mushrooms and plants to maintain health. Seeing that more and more people around the world are suffering from cancer, they drew attention to the enormous healing potential of mushrooms in this field. During their habitual nature walks, they began to focus their attention on mushrooms and plants in the forest and began to test the effects of these products on themselves. Than they started poring through literature and scientific data about the use of various types of fungi as alternative methods to treat various diseases, the result of which was this work. The world of mushrooms is huge and diverse. This book covers their tiny part.

Eugene & Svetlana Poltavets have also recently completed a larger and more comprehensive book with more detail on therapeutic uses of mushrooms and other fungi.

Medicinal Mushrooms of the Holarctic: anti-cancer & other therapeutic uses
is available from Hancock House Publishers.

More than 60 families, about 300 species of healing mushrooms
Includes Properties, Use & Preparations

SVETLANA POLTAVETS
EUGENE POLTAVETS

MEDICINAL
MUSHROOMS
OF THE HOLARCTIC

ANTI-CANCER & OTHER THERAPEUTIC USES

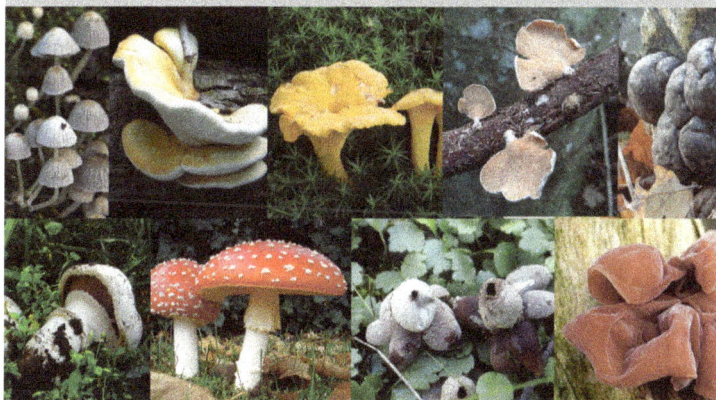

Covering ~300 species of medicinal fungi with restorative health benefits and tonic effects on the immune system, including many which possess anti-tumor properties. Also covers those species wich can help in the recovery of serious illnesses through strengthening of the immune system. Includes aspects of identification, ecology, harvest and preparation. One of the most comprehensive books of its type for the Holarctic region.

other Pacific Northwest titles from **HANCOCK HOUSE PUBLISHERS**

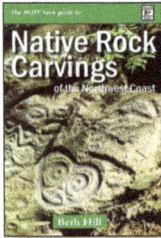

Native Rock Carvings
Beth Hill
9780888397379
5½ x 8½, sc, 48 pp
$6.95

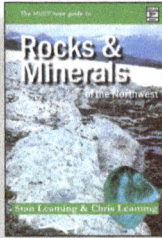

Rocks & Minerals
Stan Leaming
9780888390530
5½ x 8½, sc, 32 pp
$5.95

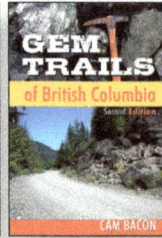

Gem Trails of BC
Cam Bacon
978-0-88839-724-9
5½ x 8½, sc, 104 pp
$12.95

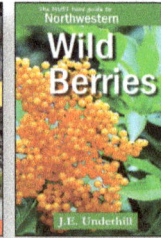

Wild Berries
J.E. Underhill
978-0-88839-027-1
5½ x 8½, sc, 96 pp
$15.95

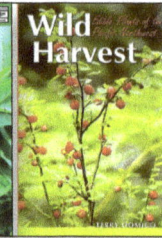

Wild Harvest
Terry Domico
978-0-88839-022-6
5½ x 8½, sc, 88pp
$14.95

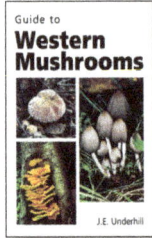

Western Mushrooms
J.E. Underhill
978-0-88839-031-8
5½ x 8½ sc, 32 pp
$5.95

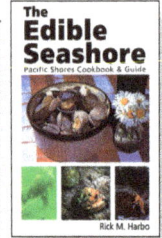

Edible Seashore
Rick Harbo
978-0-88839-199-5
5½ x 8½ sc, 62pp
$12.95

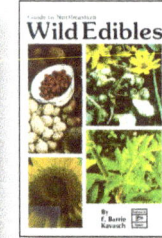

Northeastern Wild Edibles
E. Kavasch
978-0-88839-090-5
5½ x 8½ sc, 60 pp
$12.95

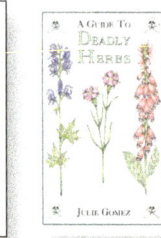

Deadly Herbs
Julie Gomez
978-0-88839-397-5
5½ x 8½, sc, 64 pp
$12.95

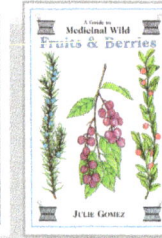

Medicinal Fruits & Berries
Julie Gomez
978-0-88839-445-3
5½ x 8½ sc, 96 pp
$12.95

Wilderness Tracks
9780888394101
5½ x 8½, sc, 72 pp
$14.95

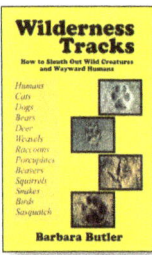

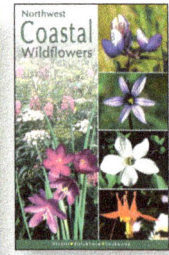

12 Basic Skills of Fly Flishing
Ted Peck
9780888393920
5½ x 8½, sc, 42pp
$11.95

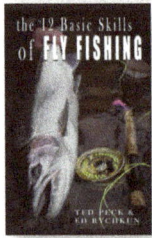

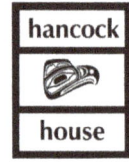

Northwest Coastal Wildflowers
978-0-88839-518-4
5½ x 8½, sc, 96 pp
$9.95

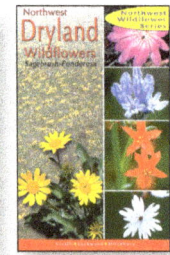

Northwest Dryland Wildflowers
978-0-88839-517-4
5½ x 8½, sc, 96 pp
$9.95

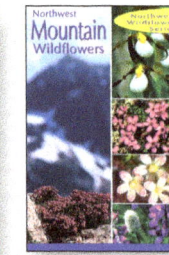

Northwest Mountain Wildflowers
978-0-88839-516-0
5½ x 8½ sc, 96 pp
$9.95

hancock house

Hancock House Publishers
www.hancockhouse.com
sales@hancockhouse.com
1-800-938-1114